M000208474

Kelsi,

Celebrate
Life!

Marcello

CELEBRATE LIFE

CELEBRATE LIFE

How to live it up, discover fulfillment,
and experience the joy you deserve.

MARCELLO PEDALINO

Copyright © 2015 by Marcello Pedalino

The right of Marcello Pedalino to be identified as the author of this work has been asserted by them in accordance with the Copyright, Designs and Patents Act 1988.

ISBN: 978-1-78324-029-6

All rights reserved. Apart from any use permitted under USA copyright law, this publication may not be reproduced, stored or transmitted by any means, without prior permission of the copyright holder/publisher.

Whilst every effort has been made to ensure that the information contained within this book is correct at the time of going to press, the author and publisher can take no responsibility for the errors or omissions contained within.

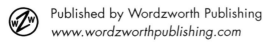
Published by Wordzworth Publishing
www.wordzworthpublishing.com

*"My father didn't tell me how to live;
he lived, and let me watch him do it."*

—CLARENCE BUDINGTON KELLAND

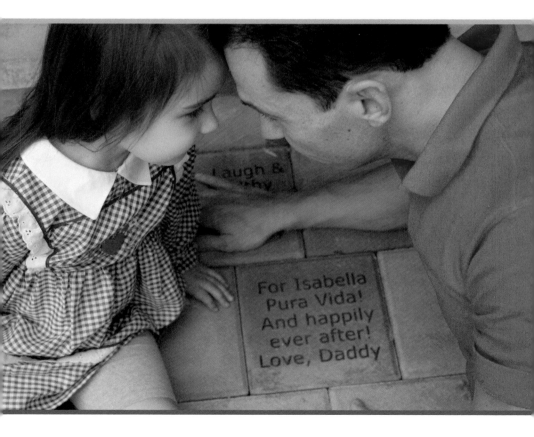

Contents

Foreword

I met Marcello Pedalino while training for my first marathon. I happened to mention that I was planning a twenty mile run and he immediately asked, "What can I do to help?" I had already mapped out a route for the run, something that would take me right along the beach the whole way (if you're going to run a twenty miler, you might as well have a nice view) but I needed a driver, someone who could take me to the start and pick me up at the end. And if that driver could also meet me every five miles and have some water and a power bar for me, that would be the icing on the cake. I explained that all to Marcello and without pause he asked, "What time do you need me?"

It was raining hard on the morning of the run. In fact, it was so bad that I considered postponing the run, but Marcello encouraged me not to. "You should always train in the worst conditions," he said. "What if it rains on race day? Anybody can do well when things are perfect." And he was right. So I decided to run and I couldn't have asked for better support. Every five miles Marcello was not only there with supplies but he had motivational music cranking from his van and was pumping me up each time. Then he even joined me for the last leg of the run.

That story pretty much sums up who Marcello Pedalino is as a person and the type of motivation and encouragement he's given me through the years. Marcello and I are in the same industry. We attend a lot of conventions together and we actually kind of look pretty similar. It is not unusual for us to be asked if we're brothers. And sometimes people mistake one of us for the other. And I'm cool with that. There's not a better man I could be associated with (or even mistaken for). In fact, it's something I'm proud of.

That story of Marcello's support on my run is also the type of real-life inspiration you can expect from this book. Marcello doesn't care if it's raining (he's had his share of rainy days as you'll find out). His attitude is, "Let's make the best of it." And then he does. In this book, he'll teach you how to do the same. He's laid out a road map and the reader just needs to follow it. Besides his own advice, he offers great suggestions from others and includes some interesting stories as well. As I read this book I felt like I did that rainy morning. Like my good friend was there to help, to motivate, and to make sure I finished what I set out to do.

I know this book will do the same for you.

by Mike Walter

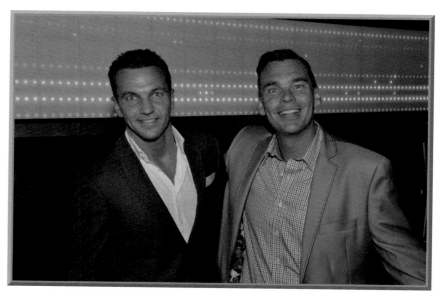

Marcello Pedalino & Mike Walter

Introduction

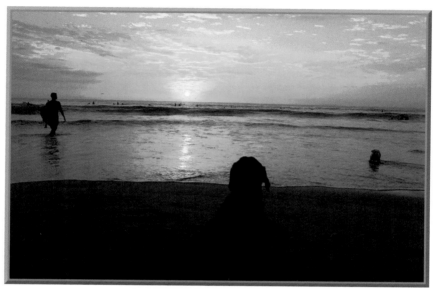

"Life should not only be lived, it should be celebrated."

—Osho

I couldn't agree more.

However, I think **waiting for someone to die so you can finally celebrate their life or waiting until you are near death to finally start celebrating your own life is absurd**. Don't get me wrong—I admire and emulate hard working people, but **waiting until you are retired to take a nice vacation, cross stuff off your bucket list, or spend more time with your family seems illogical.**

If you need a great *carpé diem* mantra as a reminder to *"seize the day,"* there are plenty of them out there already.

My friends from Costa Rica say Pura Vida, (*Pure Life*), the Jacob brothers came up with "Life is Good," and Bobby McFerrin famously sang, "Don't worry, be happy." These are all awesome and are a few of my personal favorites ... but I wanted my own. I wanted something that defined my purpose and something that was more bumper-sticker-friendly than Osho's quote to encapsulate the vibe.

About ten years ago, on a picturesque day while surfing at sunset, two words came to me as if Mother Nature whispered in my ear ... **"Celebrate Life."**

It was short and sweet, and fit my personality and purpose to a tee.

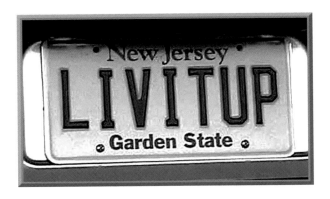

Yes, that's my license plate, and yes, that's my purpose.

What's your purpose?

Celebrate Life® is also the ideal slogan for my entertainment and event production company's brand because that's what we do. We help the world "Celebrate Life." The message was so perfect I had it registered as a Federal trademark.

The foundation of the Celebrate Life movement is built on seven key elements of wellness:

- Health
- Influence
- Lifestyle
- Adventure
- Compassion
- Wisdom
- Evolution

You can adopt and embrace this foundation as your own if you're interested in **fulfillment** like I am.

Fulfillment is the discovery of what "enough" means to you, and of course, the ultimate follow-up of actually obtaining it. Once you reach this zen-like frame of mind and attain inner peace, your celebration of life can officially begin.

And if you've never been to a party thrown by the Universe … buckle up—it's one heck of a ride to the edge of paradise!

Now don't get nervous. If that last paragraph or anything you read later sounds remotely too trippy, granola, or just a little too out there for you … rest assured that it's not. I'm as down to Earth as they come and like everybody else I appreciate **simplicity and clarity** when seeking solutions.

I don't drink, smoke, or do drugs, so no, there's never been any unnecessary influence of chemical additives either. Fortunately, I never liked the smell of cigarette smoke or the taste of alcohol. If I did, my personality type of going "all in" would have too easily lent itself to excess or addiction. I'm grateful that my desires for success, winning, and enjoying the best that life has to offer were quenched early on by my career, sports, and travel. Later in life, becoming a father and finding my true companion finally finished paving the road to fulfillment.

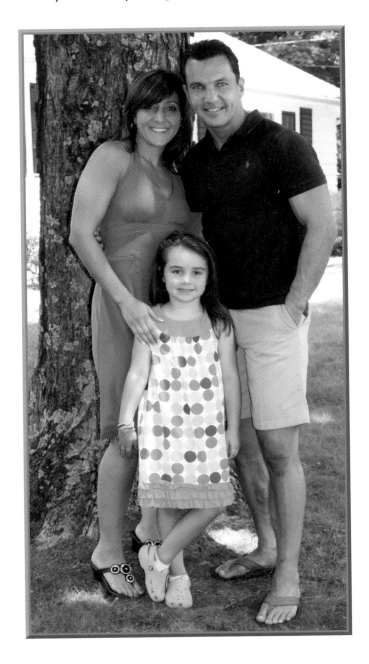

Why listen to me?

Fair question.

The answer is, you don't have to.

I was never the smartest kid in the class. Not even close. But, when someone was kind enough to slowly teach me something, or patiently show me exactly how something worked and how it should be done, I'd out-practice, out-rehearse, and out-perform everyone. I am terrible at math and all math-related subjects. But, **I know how to use a calculator and know how to make more money than I spend**. Don't ask me to point out where China is on a map. Geography and my sense of direction are embarrassing. I once ran six miles in the wrong direction after being in first place during an adventure race. But, **I learned to embrace the journey, trust my gut, and follow my heart**. I once got a concussion while jumping my bike off dirt ramps and falling on my head. I didn't have my helmet on because I didn't want to mess up my hair. But, **I aced all the classes that the school of hard knocks offered on how to survive and advance and how to endure and conquer.**

If you are already living the life that you've always wanted and you are as healthy as you should be, congratulations.

If not, read on ...

With the help of **generous family members, compassionate friends, and wise mentors,** it's taken me forty years to figure out my definition of "enough" and discover fulfillment. More times than not, I learned the hard way.

The following guidance is real and all of it has been personally road tested. **Regardless of your age, I can save you a little** (or maybe even *a lot*) of time, money, and aggravation by sharing a few of my experiences with you.

That is the purpose of this book.

Throughout the book, you'll find some noteworthy observations that have served me well called, **"Marcello's Message"**.

At the end of each chapter, you'll find a **#CelebrateLife** section that features specific action steps you can start taking immediately to **move onwards and upwards in your pursuit of fulfillment.**

A lot of good people have gone above and beyond to show me the way over the years.

It's my turn to pay it forward.

Cheers,

Marcello

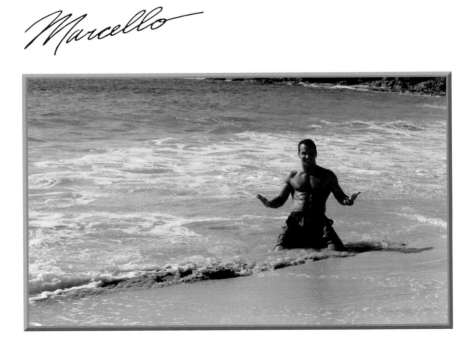

By the way, just in case you were wondering …

Is it Mar-sello**?**

or **is it** Mar-**CHELLO?**

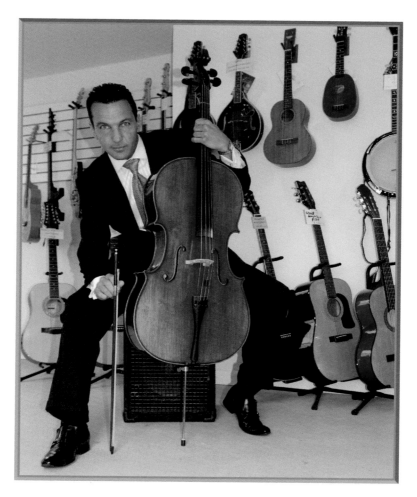

Yep. It's Mar**cello.**

CHAPTER

Take Care Of Yourself

*"Fitness can be misconstrued as being very vain
and self-centered. But it's deeper than that. You can
overcome and achieve anything with mental fortitude,
determination, and discipline."*

—FINNY AKERS

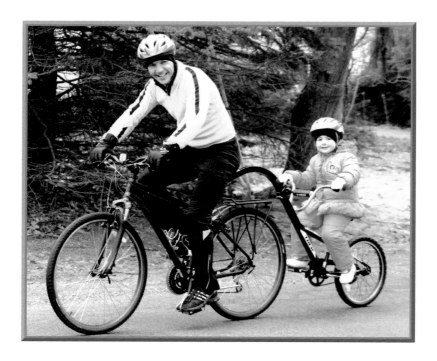

Yes, there's a good reason why wellness is first. **If you can't take care of yourself, you can't take care of your family or your clients.** In this chapter, I'll share my thoughts on exercise, nutrition, and motivation. You'll learn how an active lifestyle and eating well are non-negotiable characteristics if you want to Celebrate Life and thrive.

As a father, there's no greater fear than not being able to take care of my daughter, Isabella. Therefore, there's no greater motivation necessary. Things like being able to bike ride around the lake, water-ski, surf, build sand castles on the beach, be the cool class dad, have living room dance parties, or just run around on the playground with her are all icing on the cake.

As a business owner and marquee event host in the entertainment production and special events industry, I've said many times:

"If I look good, I feel good. If I feel good, I perform well. If I perform well, then I'll never be out of business."

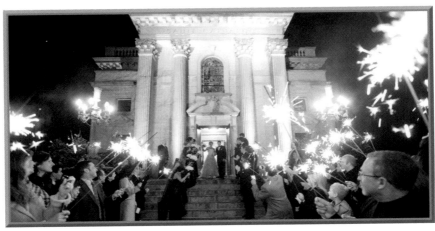

A Wedding at St. Catharine Church in Spring Lake, NJ

Whether you are the project leader or a creative partner on a signature collaboration team, maintaining optimal health and peak conditioning should be a company-wide priority. The motivation here is straightforward ... **If you want to consistently deliver exceptional service and the finest quality product to your clients, "success" and "winning" will ultimately depend on your ability to stay healthy and in the game.** You can delegate a lot of things for maximum productivity and efficiency while working—but things like your cholesterol, blood pressure, and stress levels aren't on the list.

Marcello's Message

Most entrepreneurs are taught that finding a good lawyer and a proficient accountant should be the first priority when you decide to start a company. Finding a top notch doctor and a stellar nutritionist should be added to your roster of vital team members. (*A supportive spouse or significant other is also crucial, but that's a whole other book.*)

You'll learn from most successful entrepreneurs that they're either already in the best shape possible or making the effort to re-prioritize their life and *make it happen.*

When Fortune Magazine interviewed six of the fittest CEOs in the world, they all agreed that a wellness program was paramount. Thomas Pickens from BP International is spot on. *"When you're young, fitness is sport. As you age, it's necessity ... I'm convinced that workouts not only strengthen my body but they also strengthen my mind. I never feel overwhelmed, and I rarely feel tired despite one of the toughest business schedules I've ever had."*

And not only do I love his fashion designs, I agree with Giorgio Armani's take on wellness. *"A well-maintained physique is a great business card. Ideas and intelligence are what matters, but if you have a well-maintained physique, it's better. It's a classic ideal: healthy mind, healthy body. And at least for me, discipline. Keeping the body in shape requires effort. It's the antidote to laziness, which is what I hate most of all."*

The road to **wellness starts with the food you eat**. I could've done a whole chapter on nutrition but **I'm pretty sure you already know how important it is and that you're also sick of hearing about it.**

Well, tough noogies …

Marcello's Message

If you eat out more than you do at home,
if you don't pay attention to your portions,
and you still think you can eat like you did when
you were younger without penalty,
you're making life harder than it needs to be.

And, if you really want to make things harder, do what I used to do. Eat to make yourself feel better.

There's a huge difference between going out for a nice dinner to celebrate a special occasion and going out for some comfort food to temporarily numb the pain of a rough day. Most people cross the line. In my case, the line was blurred on too many occasions. Mercifully, my physical activity level offset any moments of temporary weakness.

If you don't already know about "emotional eating," and how food intake and stress levels can go hand in hand to create a vicious cycle of depression, do yourself a favor and look into it.

Too lazy to look into it right now?

Fine.

According to medical author, Dr. Roxanne Dryden-Edwards, "Warning signs for emotional eating include a tendency to feel hunger intensely and all of a sudden, rather than gradually as occurs with a true physical need to eat that is caused by an empty stomach. Emotional eaters tend to crave junk foods rather than seeking to eat balanced meals and the urge to eat is usually preceded by stress or an uncomfortable emotion of some kind, like boredom, sadness, anger, guilt, or frustration. Another hallmark of emotional eating is that the sufferer often feels guilty for what they have eaten."

When I am asked to give seminars about Life Balance and the topic of nutrition comes up, I use the example of going through the drive-through at a Burger King. I compare it to having a one night stand. "It usually feels pretty good while you're doing it, but the next day … not so much."

The attendees always laugh at the joke because it's a funny line, but the sting of its accuracy isn't far behind.

Do you like eating waffles with bacon and Frosted Flakes for breakfast?

Do you like eating a big sandwich stacked high with deli meats and a bag of Doritos for lunch?

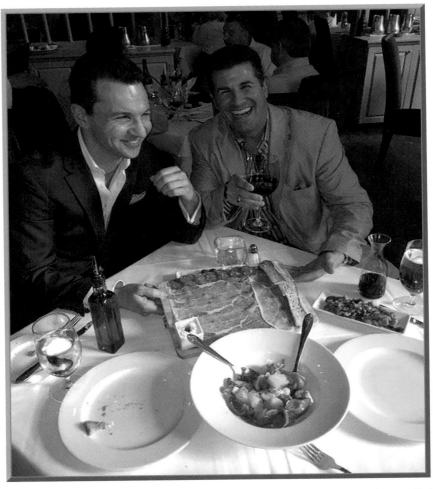

With Anthony Vennera at Davios Steakhouse in Philadelphia, PA

Do you like eating fettuccini alfredo for dinner?

I do!

Do I still eat like that every day of the week?

No way!

I love pizza, bacon cheeseburgers, pasta, bread, fresh moz-zarella, thick and juicy steaks, taylor ham, and plenty of other delicious dishes more than anyone, but I learned how to offset all those extra calories with exercise and how to spread out the gluttony over the course of a month. I learned that **if you are burning the calories, you can still enjoy a "treat" or "cheat meal" once or twice per week.** I also learned that **one of the worst things you can do is unrealistically deprive yourself from life's deliciousness.** The key is to **be aware of your weaknesses.** After you discover your weaknesses, you can find the solutions. The fixes might be a tad non-conventional, but who cares.

I never thought I'd be carrying a blender with me everywhere I go to make protein shakes in between meals to avoid snacking on Hostess CupCakes or to prevent me from going through that glorious drive-thru at Burger King. *I gave up fast food and soda years ago.*

I never thought I'd be drinking so much water that I'd pretty much have to go to the bathroom every two hours.

The numbers don't lie. A forty point drop in bad cholesterol between 36 and 39-years-old was all I needed to see to justify some notable lifestyle adjustments.

Marcello's Message

When it comes to nutrition and exercise, until a person is sick and tired of being sick and tired, they're not ready to listen to well-intended guidance and to make their personal wellness a priority.

Can you honestly say that you're as healthy as you'd like to be?

If so, good for you. If not, read on ...

It took a back injury for me to appreciate the benefits and stop making fun of people who did yoga, swam several times a week, consistently slept upwards of eight hours, paid closer attention to what they ate, and recognized the importance of

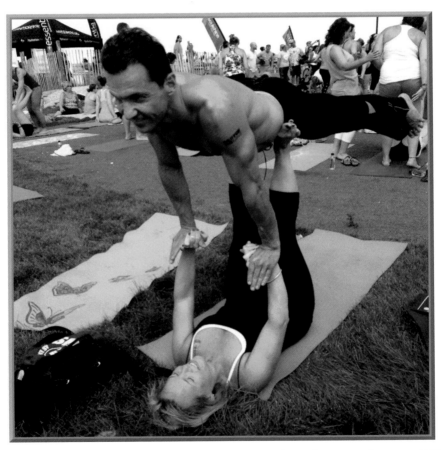

With Kelly O'Neil-Walter in Asbury, NJ

stress management. (see Chapter 6) You can experience all the glory without the pain of a hospital visit by prioritizing and finding a spot for these activities and habits in your personal wellness routine.

If nothing else, take a yoga class just once to hear the Namaste prayer that the instructor does at the end of class after *Savasana*. (A 'Corpse' pose where you lie on your back and basically take a lovely meditative nap for five minutes).

"May you find peace in your heart, peace in your home, and peace in the world."

I challenge you not to feel better about yourself and your surroundings when you walk out of there.

If for some reason you're still just as cranky, tired, and bitter towards yourself and the world in general, you better check your pulse and then immediately seek professional help because you've most likely got some deeper issues going on that need to be worked out.

Marcello's Message

If you're like me, you'll get over all of your preconceived notions and hesitations after your first experience and realize that while yoga has tremendous physical benefits, the stress-reducing benefits of being forced to slow down, regroup, and refocus for an hour are priceless.

At some point you'll need to start thinking long-term. Activities such as swimming, yoga, and hiking can be done effectively at any age. **If you want to be active into your 80s, 90s, and beyond ...** don't wait until your hips and knees need replacement, for your back to be habitually sore, or to be suffering from severe arthritis to **start doing rejuvenating full-body workouts that are gentler on the joints.**

I plan to continue to be active and enjoy a high quality of life for a long time. Pushing around a walker, with tennis balls on the bottom of it, in some nursing home with the posture of a hunchback waiting for Wheel of Fortune to come on isn't what I have in mind.

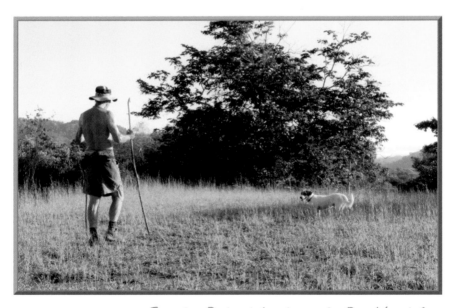

Friends: Richard Limehouse & Pee Wee hiking in Hermosa Hills, Costa Rica

#CelebrateLife

1 Get a subscription to Men's Health. The monthly content is generally uni-sex and full of helpful articles and resources. You'll get to know guys like Joe Dowdell who is a trainer, gym owner, and restaurateur who constantly shares the latest ways to improve your daily wellness routine.

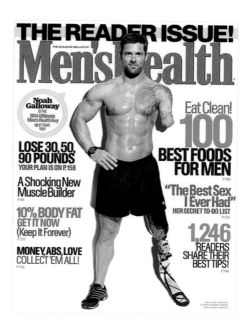

Like everything else these days, "they have an app for that" and you can get a bunch of great stuff onto your mobile device. However, I'm a firm believer that seeing an actual magazine on your coffee table, desk, or nightstand everyday versus being buried behind a screen that is loaded with an infinite number of distractions will yield a higher probability of staying focused. That being said, **when you get on a roll and reach that highly recommended sweet spot of disciplined engagement, feel free to treat yourself to all that modern technology has to offer.** *Which is a LOT of great stuff.*

2 Find a quote that feeds you a little slice of humble pie or gives you a swift kick in the butt to move onwards and upwards.

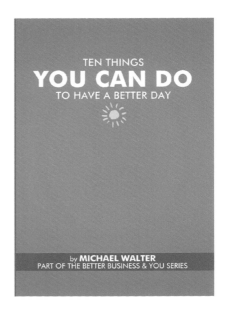

For me, at 36-years-old, the motivational quote came via my best friend, **Mike Walter.** Mike is **an accomplished entre- preneur, writer, avid con- versationalist, influential possibilitarian**, and pri- mary VIP. (see Chapter 2) **One of his books, 10 Things You Can Do To Have A Better Day, was the impetus for writing this one.**

People always ask us if we are brothers. As I told everyone at his wedding, where I had the honor to be the best man, his friendship has transcended into a brotherhood for which I am grateful. It's a brotherhood based on a solid foundation of **character, strength, and class.**

Mike passed on the words, ***"The shape you're in at 40 is a good indication of the shape you'll be in the rest of your life."*** That was all I needed to hear. That quote went up on the fridge the next day and stayed there until it was ingrained in my psyche. If you're a visual learner like me, put up a corresponding photo with it as well to enhance the daily stimulus. (see Chapter 6)

3 Create a menu that's right for you, then follow it.

But first, schedule an appointment with your doctor and get a physical to find out if you have any special medical needs or concerns. Then get your doctor's recommendation for a nutritionist to ensure that any special dietary obstacles can be addressed.

Until it becomes second nature, the menu will act as a simple and effective reminder of what to eat and when to eat it. After a month of eating properly, the nutritional choices will become second nature and you can start adding variety to keep things interesting.

Even though I'm now pretty good about knowing what to eat and when to eat it, I like having the reminder on the refrigerator. It reminds me how I should be eating if I ever get slightly off track.

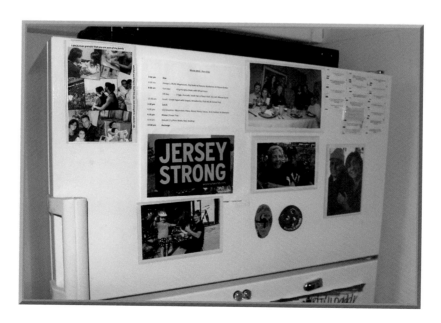

Here's a sample menu of mine:

6:00 am	Rise
6:10 am	Omega 3 capsule, Centrum multi-vitamin capsule, magnesium citrate capsule. 30g Chocolate protein shake with banana, cinnamon, frozen blueberries, and peanut butter.
9:00 am	Gym day (post workout). 42g protein shake with wheat grass. Off day: Three eggs, avocado, steak tips, sea salt, minced garlic, and ½ yam or Ezekiel English muffin.
11:30am	Snack: Greek yogurt with almonds and prunes.
1:30pm	Lunch: Chicken, turkey, London broil, tuna fish or sweet Italian sausage over a spring mix salad.
3:15pm	**Refresh**: Run, bike, or kayak.
4:00pm	25g protein shake with a dash of maca, dash of macai, honey, dash of cacau, dash of acai, and a dash of quinoa. Green tea with honey.
6:30pm	Dinner: Salmon, tilapia, pork loin, soup or sushi with asparagus, broccoli or edamamme with brown rice and quinoa.
9:30pm	**Rebuild**: 25g protein shake, bed, reading.
10:00pm	**Recharge:** Lights out.

4. Use this simple and clever line from Adelle Davis, known by many as "The first lady of nutrition," if you're not sure how much to eat during the day. ***"Eat breakfast like a King, lunch like a Prince, and dinner like a pauper."*** Just because you may have been blessed with good appetite and a good metabolism, it doesn't mean you should have that third slice of pizza or that second bowl of pasta. I learned that **just because you can, doesn't mean you should.** This is when water comes in handy. Drink a big glass and wait for fifteen minutes ... you might surprise yourself how the hunger magically disappears.

5. Make the next Marcello's Message one of your daily mantras if you can't stick with a wellness upgrade attempt;

> ### Marcello's Message
>
> It's easier to stay in shape than it is to get back into shape ... consistency is key.

Strength and conditioning coach, Matthew Ibrahim, wraps it up nicely ...

"The important point here is that in order to remain healthy and out of the pain cave, it's an absolute requisite for you to bulletproof your body with some prehab-rehab exercises in order to decrease the likelihood of injury. It's near impossible to stay injury-free forever, but using an effective and efficient program that targets your weakest points will minimize the likelihood of injury, and even limit the severity of injuries if and when they do occur ... Everyone will get

their usual aches and pains along the way to training hard and training passionately, but the real goal is to avoid the big hurdles that keep us on the shelf and out of the gym for prolonged periods of time. Ultimately, the break in routine and the inability to train uninhibited will get in the way of our ability to make progress towards our goals on a consistent basis."

6 **Here are a few of my favorite *healthier*-than-hostess-Cup-Cakes-snacks that you might also enjoy**:

- Popcorn followed by watermelon.
- Kale chips followed by grapes or strawberries.
- Grannie Smith apple with almond butter.
- 2 slices of turkey and hummus wrapped in a slice of Swiss cheese.
- 1 hardboiled egg wrapped in 2 slices of roast beef.
- Handful of almonds and 2 prunes followed by an orange.

7 If you miss having pancakes drizzled with syrup, like I do, try some quick and healthy pan-crepes drizzled with agave instead. *(Mix up two eggs, one banana, and two dashes of cinnamon. Serve with fresh strawberries and a tall glass of orange juice.)* This is our go-to breakfast after a nice Sunday morning workout.

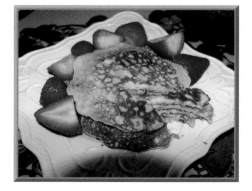

8 **And that trick you may have heard about?** When you order something like a chicken parmesan and spaghetti dinner from a restaurant and it's a huge portion, divide it in half and ask your server to immediately wrap up the other half in a "to go" container so you don't unnecessarily over-eat …

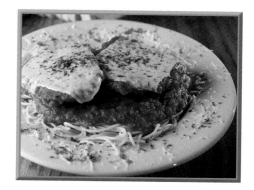

Yes, it works

… and, you've got lunch for the next day.

CHAPTER
Keep Good Company

2

"The fastest way to change yourself is to hang out with people who are already the way you want to be."

—REID HOFFMAN

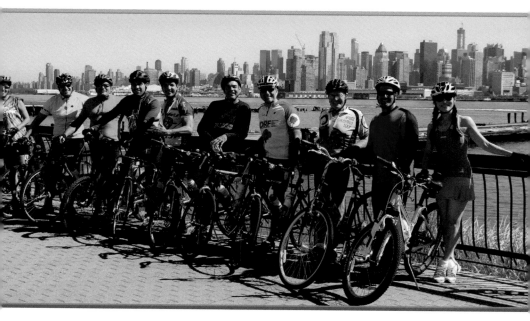

In Jersey City on the annual Celebrate Life Ride

From left: Betsy Fischer, Anthony Vennera, George Panzitta, Jack Bermeo, Marcello Pedalino, Mike Walter, John DeRienzo, Tony Shaughnessy, Dave Nase, & Baiju Wang

When your health and wellness become a priority, you'll soon learn that the people you hang around with are a key ingredient to staying on track. In this chapter, I'll introduce you to a few of the many inspirational people in my life, and tell you how to start surrounding yourself with positive influences.

I've been a big fan of my fabulous Aussie friend, rock star speaker, and super productivity expert, Neen James, since the day she schooled me on what she calls **Conscious Celebration.** *You don't have the time to do everything, you only have time to do what matters.* Right on! Any time I'm faced with a tough choice in my daily schedule between doing just one activity instead of multiple options, I think of Neen's wise words and proceed accordingly.

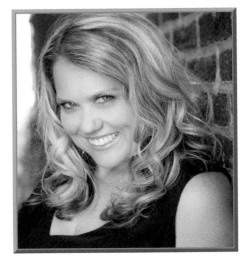

Neen James

After a few lunches with Neen, I also learned there are two different types of people in this world.

VIPs and VDPs

VIPs are Very Inspiring People. They make you laugh, think, and ponder notable possibilities. **They help you help yourself, but always offer support when you can't.** They tell you things that make you feel good about yourself when you've earned the praise but also tell you the truth when you fall short—without hesitation ... which many times is not easy on the ears.

Marcello's Message

A friend is someone who tells you what you want to hear. A good friend is someone who tells you what you need to hear.

They respect your time and circumstances. They know how to relax as much as they are gritty workhorses, but will always remind you that "**complacency is the enemy of progress.**"

Your childhood friends are a great source for VIP prospecting. I still play poker and go out to dinner frequently with the same guys I hung out with in the 8th grade.

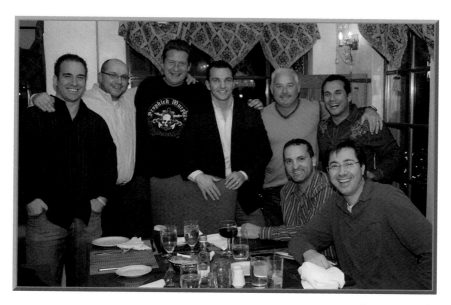

Oakland, NJ

From top left: Jim Reckenbeil, Sasa Trajkovic, Brian Florence, Marcello Pedalino, Tommy Few, Gabe Savarese

From bottom left: Jason Sammarco & Berendt Gugleberger

These guys are **brutally honest**, hysterical, and always make sure that you keep your ego in check. *Especially when they see another complimentary article about your business or another personal accolade online using your fancy Italian nickname.*

VIPs are **possibilitarians**. **They don't preach opinionated rhetoric or speak in absolutes; instead they encourage fact-based dialogue without prejudice or limitations.** They wear rose-colored glasses but they're realists. **They like rainbows and butterflies but know that reality bites sometimes.**

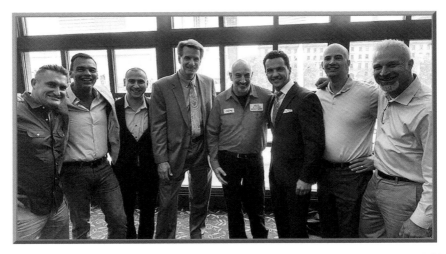

Clevelend, OH

From left: Jason Jani, Mike Walter, Matt Radicelli, Jim Cerone, Jeffrey Gitomer, Marcello Pedalino, Beau Kramer & Adrian Cavlan

Moreover, many possibilitarians are very witty and have a gloriously dry sense of humor to boot.

Folks like Mike even tune in to the fictional radio station that we created called **WKIP** *(We Keep It Positive).* It was put on air for all the times that life kicks your butt. **The listener's job**

is to find the good, no matter how bad it just went down. This is when the ability to stay calm and offer levity via sarcastic, dark, and snarky comments comes in handy.

Marcello's Message
You are who you surround yourself with.

The special events industry is filled with VIPs. I'm very fortunate and grateful to call many of them dear friends.

Randy Bartlett is a **supremely talented Master of Ceremonies** trainer, and a connoisseur of humor and levity. He also has a way with timing and the spoken word. Earlier in my career, I remember hearing him say four words at one of his seminars that had a huge impact on my personal and professional development, ***"Work less. Live More."*** He was talking about the business model that I adopted soon

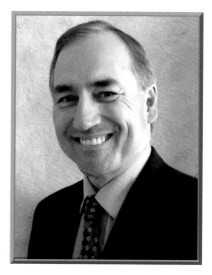

Randy Bartlett

after. Essentially, when you work, work your tail off, and work for people that have the means to appreciate it so you can actually go out and enjoy the fruits of your labor. (see Chapter 3) Randy's influence was also the reason I knew that making a few hundred thousand dollars more each year, but having to work eighteen hours a day and hardly sleeping would never be worth it.

Jason Jani is **a marquee mixologist and event producer** who deserves all of the industry recognition he gets for being **creative, innovative, and putting in the hustle every day.**

His philosophy is …

"If you lack creativity and can't think outside the box, you will simply live in the average. Average has never been good enough for me, or my business. That's my motivation every day. Do something good. Be original. Be awesome. ***Make it happen."***

Before I even knew what a hashtag was, he already made the **#MakeItHappen** hashtag well known in the special events world. Similar to Nike's old ad campaign, "Just Do It." "Make it Happen" **are three words that have become a crucial chant when I'm teetering on making excuses instead of results.**

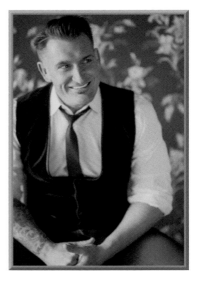

Jason Jani

Jason also turned me on to Gary Vaynerchuk and the joys of "crushing it" daily. A notable daily crush could be a great workout, annihilating your to-do list, or just emptying your inbox. *Sometimes I get just as excited about cleaning the house, washing the cars, doing the laundry, or cooking a delicious family dinner.* Seeing how much I can accomplish in a day without sacrificing quality or leisure activities is a very fun and productive game to play.

From an entertainment and production standpoint, a special event can be crushed as well. Signature collaborations with Jason and his team have enabled me to evolve professionally from a DJ to an event host and producer. Our potent blend of talent, production elements, and mutual quest for perfection have yielded spectacular celebrations and very happy clients.

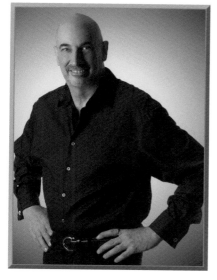

Jeffrey Gitomer

Jeffrey Gitomer is one of my favorite writers and professional speakers. He created a really simple formula that constantly reminds me that knowledge without action is wasted potential.

He wrote,
"Knowing + Doing = Living."

Whenever I see this, I cringe and remember all the time I used to waste watching too much television—especially late at night before I learned the importance getting to bed early and getting up early. It was usually around 2 am and by default I'd be watching a cheesy self-help infomercial that came on after the cool movie I was watching was over. *(By the way, do you know what's worse than staying up way too late to watch a movie when you should be sleeping? Staying up way too late to watch a movie that you already have on DVD that you could watch at any time … without commercials!)* I remember thinking that the advertiser's product and words might actually work for any bleary-eyed viewer and help them make their life better, **(Knowing)** but if the viewer doesn't get their butt up off the couch, **(Doing)** the self-imposed rat race finish line will never be crossed. **(Living)**

I remember coming to the embarrassing realization that watching television at 2 am wasn't **doing** anything but making it harder to wake up the next day to work out and be productive.

Gitomer also knows that couples have plenty of other viable options for entertainment before going to bed than staring at a television. *This is where having the right spouse or significant other comes into play again.*

Marcello's Message

There's nothing wrong with watching a show for a few laughs, catching the big game, or watching a superb documentary, but remember that T.V. is like food—moderation is key.

Most social media platforms share a similar potential death spiral and should be treated as such. **Have you ever gone on YouTube to watch a funny skit by Jimmy Fallon only to find yourself forty three minutes later watching classic music videos from the 80s and clips of people doing some magnificently-stupid things?**

I have.

VDPs are Very Draining People.

Can you think of anyone in your life who can come up with a problem for every solution? Me, too. **That's a VDP.**

Like kryptonite for Superman, **a VDP is anyone in the world who is holding you back from your pursuit of fulfillment.** Beware, they come in all shapes and sizes, and unfortunately some can actually be people with whom you share an intimate relationship or significant friendship.

Marcello's Message

One of the hardest lessons I learned was that people change ... and not always for the better. Growth is usually a good thing, but understand that growing apart is always a possibility.

There's an **outstanding keynote speaker** named Bryan Dodge who tours the convention and corporate training circuit. His word for a VDP is a **"Bad Seed."** He says when you see someone who is just oozing unconstructive or negative mojo, reach out your hands like you are zapping them and say *"Bad Seed! Bad Seed!"* and run the other

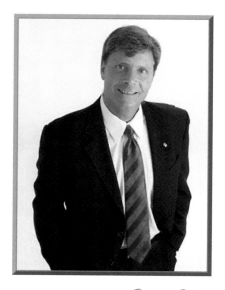

Bryan Dodge

way. First, this will make you giggle *(which is always a good thing)*, and then they'll probably think you're nuts so they won't bother you anymore. Unless you are in prison, and locked up with someone, there is no reason to stay in the presence of a VDP who is making your life miserable or less gratifying than you deserve.

Many people have asked me over the years how I maintain such a positive attitude. It's simple. I have a very low tolerance for mean people and negativity. Bryan's funny yet effective way to handle them works like a charm every time.

Before you go dismissing many of the people you'll encounter on a daily basis, know that everyone has a bad day and they might be experiencing some challenging circumstances behind the scenes. Try not to judge too quickly. As you get older and wiser, and talk to people with more experience than you, who have dealt with this kind of nonsense, you'll eventually learn when to "say when" and to trust your gut.

#CelebrateLife

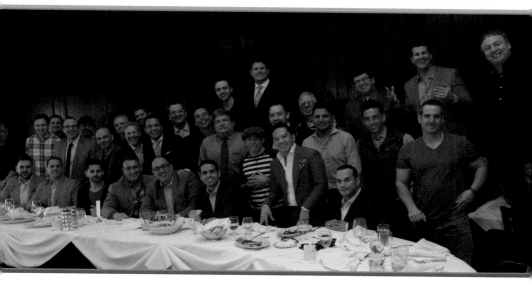

A Celebrate Life Luncheon "For The Gentlemen" at Maggiano's.

Standing from left: Michael Chieffo, Chris D'Amico, Michael "Bird" McHugh, Jimmy Mousouroulis, Joe Falco, Lorenzo Araneo, Tony Tee Neto, Sean "Big Daddy" McKee, John Murphy, Paul Knox, Marcello Pedalino, Izzy Feliu, Mike Walter, George Panzitta, Strato Doumanis, Jeffrey Scott Gould, Bobby Carpenter, Jack Bermeo, Ble Hamilton Yalong, Jonny Dee, Edson Munroy, Erik Kent, Paul Anthony Centamore, Anthony Vennera, Dave Nase, Sir Paul Evan

Sitting from left: Josh Christie, Joey Di Pietro, Tony Gia, Jason Jani, Gerlando Siracusa, Vincent Velasquez & Gabe Savarese

1   **Remove yourself** *(gracefully and respectfully when possible)* **from the company of negative influences and detrimental situations** both at home and at work. **Don't look back.**

2   Write down the names of the people in your immediate circle of influence. Note which ones are **driven, passionate, gracious, and worldly**. Reach out to every one of them. First, **say "thank you," and be specific for the reason.** Then, wait. You'll be surprised who actually takes the time to respond. Whoever does, with more than just a "yeah, I know I'm awesome" and actually acknowledges your good intentions, will **make your short-list of where to cultivate your new surroundings** in the near future. **Pretty easy.**

CHAPTER 3

Do What You Love

"Never continue in a job you don't enjoy. If you're happy in what you're doing, you'll like yourself, you'll have inner peace. And if you have that, along with physical health, you will have had more success than you could possibly have imagined."

—JOHNNY CARSON

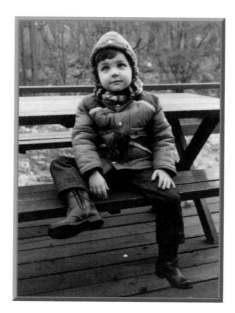

Oakland, 1978

Often times, you will find yourself at home or work staring off into the distance and pondering the popular question that many overachievers and type A personalities ponder from time-to-time … **"is this as good as it gets?"**

While consistent introspection is a necessary evil to gauge whether or not you need to make a move, be careful not to lose the magical peace of mind that comes with the ability to live in the present and be grateful for what you have. Like the title of the classic song by John Lennon and Paul McCartney, and the content of this chapter, the discovery of doing what you love is sometimes A Long and Winding Road. In this chapter, I'll introduce you to my family and share the moves I made along my journey. I'll tell you why listening to your parents is usually a good idea and how time will always be more valuable than money. You'll learn how to pursue a fulfilling career that you're passionate about and the power of re-prioritizing your life.

Marcello's Message

If you love to use the expression **"It is what it is"** like I used to, the chances of you *allowing* mediocrity in your life go up exponentially. *Never* settle until all options have been explored and exhausted.

My personal journey began at home …

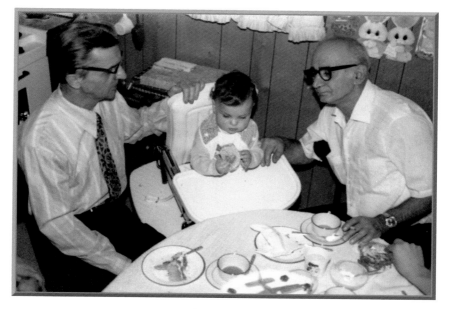

With Grandpa Julius Csepela (left) and Grandpa Victor Pedalino (right) in Belleville, NJ 1974

Grandpa Julius (from the Irish and Hungarian side of the family) used to get all the slightly dented soup cans and day-old bread for free from the grocery store. He gave me a big bag of assorted and individually wrapped candy to enjoy when I was a junior in high school. I liked candy, but I wasn't going to eat 150 pieces. I took the candy to school and sold it to my classmates. **I learned three important things that day:**

1 I could make a lot of money.

2 **I could make a lot of people happy.**

3 I could make a lot of money while **making a lot of people happy AND have a lot of fun.**

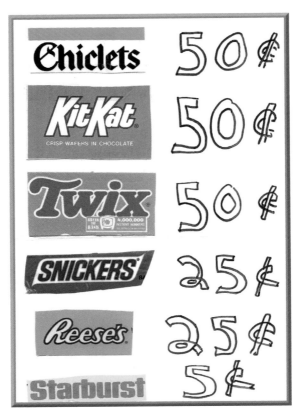

*The "Candyman's" homemade pricing menu
for the candy business, Indian Hills High
School, 1989*

It wasn't long before I had the candy manufacturers delivering wholesale cases of candy to my house and a little section of my parents' basement became a makeshift warehouse. I made a $6000 net profit by the end of the year. **The faculty and administrators** (most of whom were regular customers) **eventually wised up and installed vending machines filled with candy so the money could go towards the school** instead of "The Candyman", as I was known by my classmates.

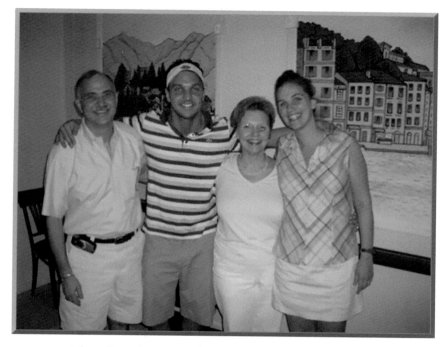

With Dad—Victor, Mom—Tracy, and sister—Sharmon, 2005

My parents were always supportive of all my little entrepreneurial endeavors and **are my greatest influencers**. Even in their retirement, they continue to lead by example and teach me the importance of **hard work, compassion, gratitude, staying in touch** with family and old friends, and of course, **having fun.**

A student of Dale Carnegie, **Mom** was the **consummate saleswoman** who always knew how to channel her inner Emily Post and Jackie O. Handwritten thank you notes and seemingly effortless **hospitality, style, and grace** were her forte.

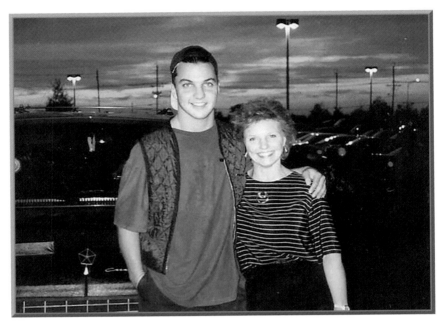

With mom in Stanhope, 1993

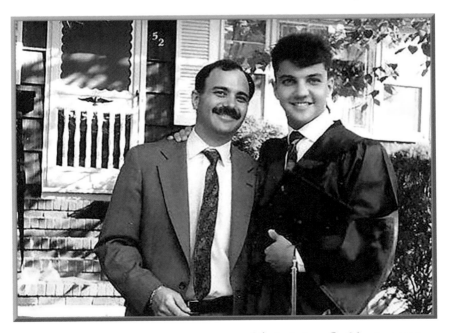

With dad in Oakland, 1991

Dad was a special agent in the DEA whose **street-smarts, tenacity, charisma**, and **logistical savvy** enabled him to have a decorated career as well. *Think Al Pacino in Serpico.*

My older **sister** was, and still is, **athletic, intelligent, pretty**, and **loved by everyone. A warm smile is something she wears every day**.

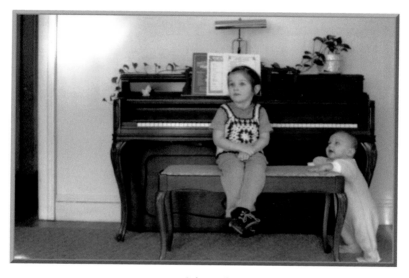

With Sharmon in Belleville, 1974

She also got our mom's sky blue eyes which, when combined with the aforementioned smile, makes for a pleasant introduction and memorable encounter.

Following two years behind her in school became a gift and a not-so-bad curse. **A lot of doors were opened because of her reputation, but it brought along a lot of pressure and desire to not only maintain the outstanding name that *she* earned, but to develop my own admirable reputation as well.** I ended up doing just fine in most of the categories ... except for the stellar grades.

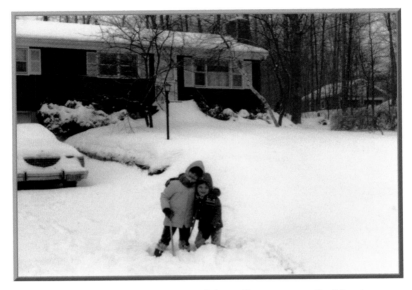

With Sharmon in Oakland, 1978

After high school, my father told me, *"You can either get a full-time job, go to college, or move out of my house."* **At the time I thought this was a *bit* harsh, but looking back, it seems like a pretty fair and reasonable ultimatum.**

Mark Twain inspired a quote that you may have also learned to appreciate over the years.

"The older you get, the smarter your parents become."

Marcello's Message

If by chance your mom or dad have gotten smarter as you've gotten older, and they're still around to hear the words, now's a good time to **put down the book** and **make a call** to say **"thanks for everything"** and **"I love you."**

Trust me, I'm no Hallmark Card groupie and I'm definitely not the mushy gushy sentimental type, but I know that **most people don't say these two phrases enough** to people they care about.

This is a perfect time to recognize Al and Lynn.

After my sister and I graduated high school, my parents decided it was best for our family for each of them to pursue a new beginning. In following their hearts, they both eventually found their true companion. Isabella and I are extremely grateful and fortunate to have Mom and Al and Dad and Lynn in our lives.

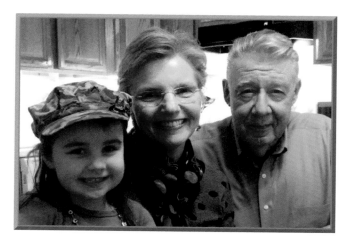

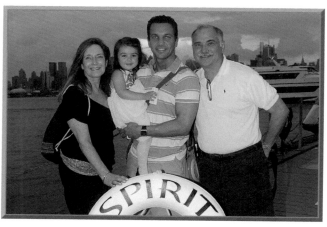

Back to the ultimatum ...

First, I chose community college. *Actually, my grades didn't give me any other choice.* **I always enjoyed writing, sociology, business administration, performing arts, and communications, but all the other prerequisite-y nonsense that was mandatory for some reason, made it nearly impossible to stay in my seat.** *That statistics professor, who didn't like to answer questions and had the personality of a brick, didn't help the cause either.*

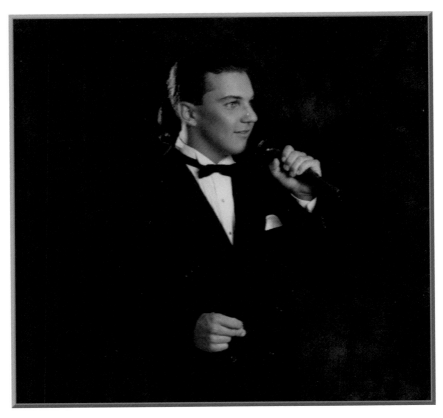

Circa 1995: When I thought Steven Seagal and his slicked-back pony tail were really cool

Then, I made the mistake of trying to take these courses during the summer when the weather forecast favored going to the beach or playing tennis instead of sitting idly in a smelly classroom.

A full time job was next on the list of options. It was for a local florist. **I enjoyed designing, manicuring, and maintaining arrangements at the shop and making airport runs to pick up exotic orchids from Hawaii.** I'm not sure why or how, but the next thing I knew my job description turned into landscaping the boss's rental properties.

Ok. I enjoyed being outdoors so why not?

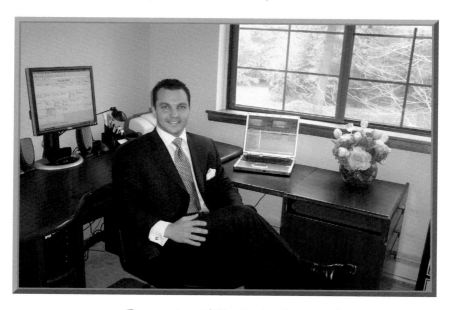

Featured in NJ's Daily Record Newspaper, 2003

One day, after spending all morning and the early afternoon hours cleaning up the yard of a house that had been neglected for quite some time, I took a break for lunch. **As I sat down to eat, my boss showed up and gave his approval for my job. I** was ready to take a bite of my sandwich and bask in the sunny glory for what should have been my *hour-long* break when he followed up with an Ebenezer Scrooge-like bark and yelled out, "Break's over in fifteen minutes. See ya back at the shop!"

That was my last day at the shop.

After learning that I told Ebenezer to "take this job and shove it," my mother put in a good word for me at the local dry-cleaner and so began my next job delivering shirts. All was going well when the manager (who knew I loved music and knew that I had invested the 6k from the candy business into some audio gear) asked me to "DJ" his brother's wedding. I happily accepted and did a pretty decent job. Much of my **attention-to-detail, perfectionist inclinations,** and **hospitality-friendly personality traits** came in handy and I booked two more milestone events from there.

When my father gave me that ultimatum of college, full time job, or moving out, my mother gave me lunch invitations with three of the most successful entrepreneurs in town. **Those lunches opened my eyes to what was possible and helped give me the courage necessary to Celebrate Life on my own terms.** The whole *working from 9-5 for someone you don't like and doing something you don't love, before and after sitting in traffic everyday waiting for a measly two week vacation-* thing was never going to happen. Everyone has his or her idea of The American Dream. **I made a deal with myself that I would live in a shack eating peanut butter and jelly sandwiches for as long as it took for my own company to prosper.** I was **"all in. "** It never got that extreme, but I got my own place soon thereafter and started *the hustle.*

Marcello's Message

Have you ever been "all in"?
Have you ever wanted something so bad that
you were willing to put your creature comforts
and safe but mind-numbing status
quo on the line for it?
When mean people do this, it's horrifying.
When good people do this, it's astounding.

Can you honestly say that you do what you love?

If not, are you at least embracing the journey?

After all the twists and turns, I'm grateful to say that I do what I love.

I help the world celebrate life.

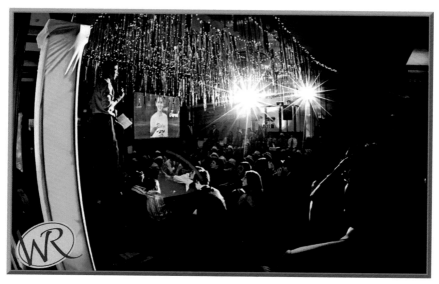

A Bar Mitzvah at the Grand Summit Hotel in Summit, NJ

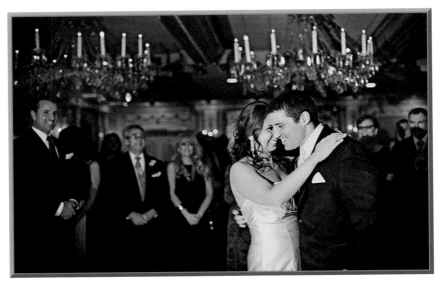

A Wedding at The Manor in West Orange, NJ

For the past twenty five years, people contact my team to help them *make it happen*.

Whether it's an exclusive corporate event in Sun Valley, Idaho, an elegant wedding reception in Palm Beach, Florida, or a fabulous Bat Mitzvah celebration in Costa Rica, we provide the **talent, lighting design, production, behind-the-scenes logistics,** and **on-site event hosting.**

My discerning clientele has high expectations, which keep me on my toes. I work with **happy people** who have gathered together to celebrate something **positive**. *It's like the opposite of working in the customer service department for the cable company or DMV.*

What's more important to you? Money, status, or time?

I work from home. I make "**enough**" **money to pay the bills and put a little away**. Most importantly, I earn "**TIME ...**" to not

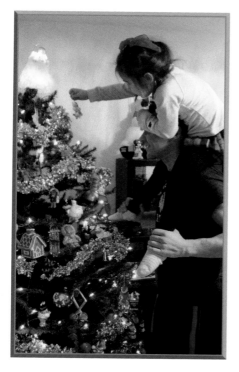

With Isabella, 2014

only eat lunch when I want and for as long as I want, but to **enjoy life's deliciousness with family and friends when it matters most.**

When Isabella was born, I lost count of how many times my mentors and parents with grown children told me to make sure that I "enjoy every moment." "Don't blink. It goes by fast," they said. "Before you know it, she'll be getting on the bus for Kindergarten. Those are the moments you'll treasure forever. Don't let the trivial things in life get in the way."

I took all those wise words to heart and made sure that work would never trump the irreplaceable memories of being there for my kid's childhood.

Marcello's Message

Always heed the advice of people who are more experienced, smarter, or better at something than you are.

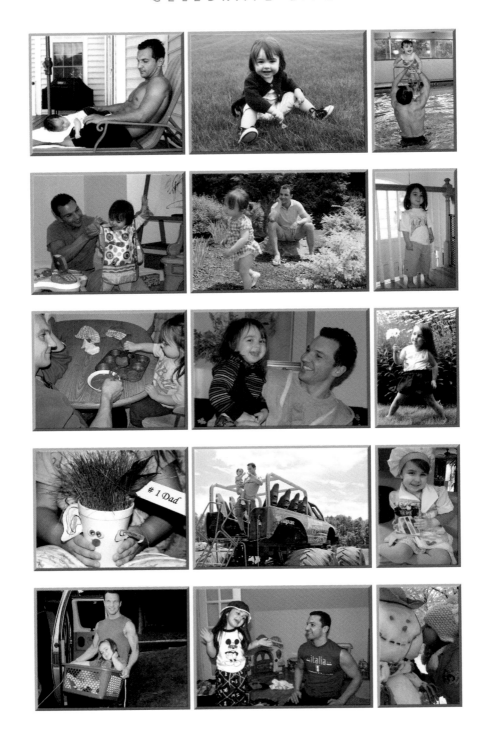

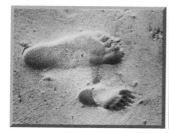
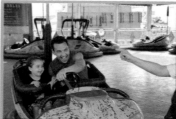
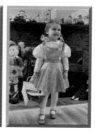

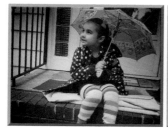
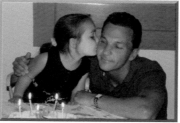
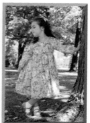

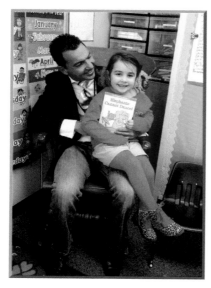
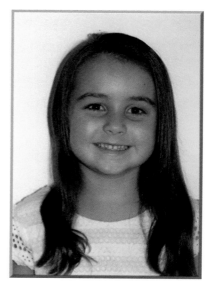

What do you think of Bentley's classic ad campaign?

"Time is life's most precious commodity,
you have to savor every second."

I love it.

I LIVE IT.

#CelebrateLife

1 Determine what makes you happy. Go do it. Not sure? Travel outside your comfort zone, both literally and geographically, (see Chapter 4) to see what piques your interest and narrow down the possibilities. Or, just go to your local library! It's a magical place that allows you to travel anywhere in the world and talk to the most brilliant minds in history without spending a dime. You could just Google an intriguing location, person, or national treasure and call it a day, but being in a library will put you in the right frame of mind to learn and open your mind without as many distractions. ** Do not bring your phone inside with you. **

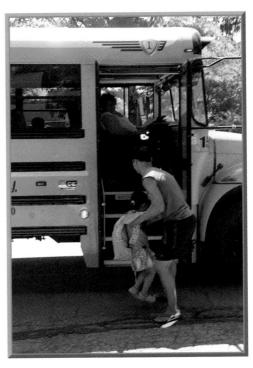

Isabella's first day of kindergarten

2 Talk to people who already love what they do. (see Chapter 2) An email or phone call is fine, but if you really want to stand out, hand-write a note and mail it.

Not sure what to say? No worries … Try something like this.

> Hi **(awesome person)**,
>
> I read one of your recent **(books/blogs/posts/ articles)** called ("_____" **include title and date)**. The part about the **(be specific)** really **(inspired me/ made me think/resonated with me.)**
>
> If your schedule permits, I'd like to take you to lunch next month. I'm trying to expand my network of really smart and talented individuals. **Plus, I just read this awesome new book called Celebrate Life by Marcello Pedalino and he told me that I should do this.** (just kidding)
>
> I've got two dates available as of now, **(Thursday the 5th at 12:30 pm or Tuesday the 17th at 1:30 pm)**. At your earliest convenience, please let me know if you are available. The best way to reach me is … **(leave your e-mail & cell phone)**
>
> Thank you for your time! Cheers!
>
> **(Your name)**

If they don't get back to you within a week, try one more time just in case the correspondence got misplaced or lost in the spam folder, etc. If you don't hear anything back the second time around … they are not a good candidate for your personal circle of influence.

3 Figure out a way to make "enough" money to support your passion and maintain a healthy soul. Ideally, become your own boss if possible. *Or, at least find a boss who is a VIP.* Chances are, they'll be more inclined to accommodate your lifestyle as long as you do your part.

Be prepared to live in a smaller house, drive an older car, and not buy as much stuff. *All of which you'll eventually find out is what you should've been doing all along anyway.* Writer *David Friedlander*, who works with LifeEdited.com creator Grahm Hill, agrees about the "luxury of less." *"Imagine you are editing the story of your life. What parts of the plot are essential? Which settings are necessary? Which characters are indispensable? And what could be left out? What parts of your life feel like filler?*

Now stop imagining, because you **are** *editing the story of your life. Every choice you make—the home you live in, the furniture you buy, the knickknacks on the mantle, the relationships you keep, the career you choose, the activities you engage in, the media you consume—shape your story …*

Your personal edit might be buying a smaller home, participating in a car share, or buying one less pair of jeans. **The specifics are not important. Simply remember that everything you add to your life that is not important, detracts from everything that is. "**

CHAPTER 4

Travel

4

"Take vacations. Go as many places as you can.
You can always make more money.
You can't always make more memories."

—via Glenn & Jenifer Roush

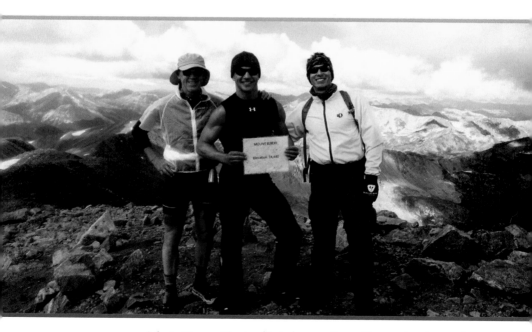

With Doug Nash (left) and Ron Michaels (right)
on the summit of Mt. Elbert, Colorado

Growing up in Jersey, it didn't take long to realize how fortunate I was to see the seasons change, to head down the shore, to go hiking in the mountains, or go have dinner and see a Broadway show in New York City. In this chapter, you'll find out that even though Dorothy was right when she said, *"there's no place like home,"* adventures abroad can have an indelible impact on your future. I'll also share some of my traveling experiences with you and show you that making it happen is easier than you think.

Marcello's Message

A trip around the world may not be in the budget and you may not have the stones to lace up your new Nike sneakers and run across the country like Forrest Gump, but fear not. Just start by getting as far away from your zip code as possible.

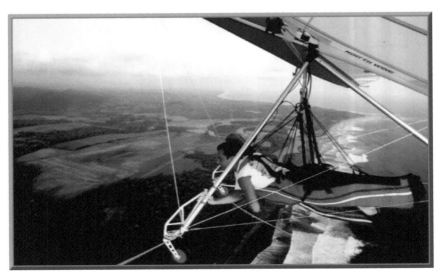

Playa Hermosa, Costa Rica

That being said, my mentors and circle of influence couldn't have been more on point when they said, *"If you really want some perspective and are hungry for some more of life's nuggets that they don't teach you in the classroom, hop on a plane and go international."*

As an avid surf-kayaker, sun worshiper, and lover of convenient direct flights out of Newark Airport, **Costa Rica soon became my home away from home during the cold and snowy northeast winters.**

Over the years, my new friends there became like family. **They re-taught me how to eat, exercise, chill out, and live by their own Celebrate Life mantra, "Pura Vida. "** (Pure Life)

This popular tag line has a bunch of different micro translations. **The two-word recipe basically boils down to a sweet melodic dish of some Namaste, Hang Loose, Hakuna Matata,**

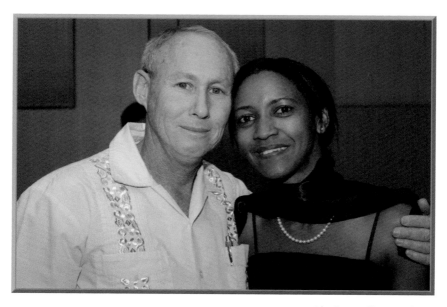

Neil & Yasmin Kahn

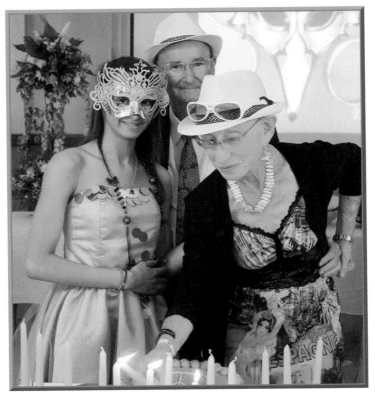

Melanie Kahn, with her grandparents, Norma & Ken

L' Chaim, and Life Is Good served up just right like Goldilocks' porridge.

Speaking of L'Chaim, the incredible Kahn family, who treat me like a son every time I'm in town, (including Shabbat dinners every Friday night), gave my company the honor of producing its first international Bat Mitzvah a few years ago.

Even more important than the lifestyle upgrade was the per-spective-rebirth that occurred when I got to know some of the Ticos (Costa Ricans) and transplanted locals. Like Jersey, I found all sorts of socioeconomic classes in Costa Rica. How-

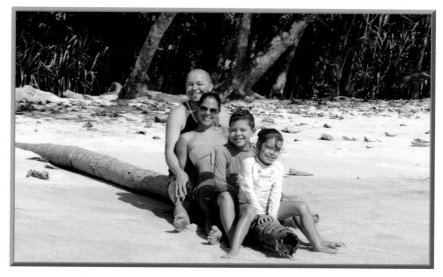

The Segura Family: Renato, Damaris, Brython & Samantha

ever, **most of the people there have half as much as we do but are twice as happy as we are.** I learned how some people, like **my friend Renato** and his family, can live a bountiful existence with only three things—family, fútbol (American Soccer), and great music. Seriously. And for my friends who surf, just add great waves to that trifecta and everybody is good to go. I think chef and author *Anthony Bourdain* sums it up nicely.

> *"Travel changes you. As you move through this life and this world you change things slightly, you leave marks behind, however small. And in return, life—and travel—leave marks on you. Most of the time, those marks—on your body or on your heart—are beautiful ..."*

When was the last time you traveled out of town for something other than work?

If it took you longer than two seconds to answer that question, it's been too long.

Marcello's Message

Everyone I've ever spoken to about their favorite memories mentions the times when they went on vacation with their parents.
If you have kids, take them with you whenever possible.
If you think working more and leaving them with more money will make them happy, you're wrong.

My parents did the best they could with what they had to give my sister and I an **awesome** childhood. They subscribed to Sam Cawthorn's philosophy, *"The happiest people don't necessarily have the best of everything but they make the most of everything."*

Summer trips down the shore will always be treasured. **Nothing fancy**—just cold cut sandwiches, the juiciest peaches, chilled

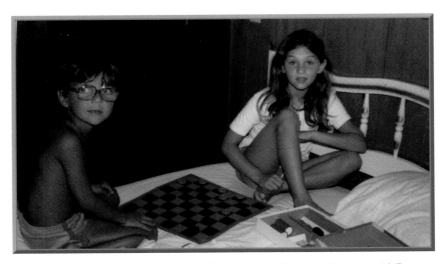

With Sharmon in Ortley Beach, NJ 1980

cans of Coca Cola, and Italian Ices on **a sunny day at the beach** with grandparents, aunts, uncles, and cousins.

We would play in the sand and waves all day, go home for a simple pasta and meatballs dinner, and then just play checkers, rummy 500, and Uno until it was time to go to bed. The next day, we'd get up and do it all over again and have **the time of our lives.**

My **beloved and extraordinary** Grandmother, "***Grandma Dora***," was **the reason I fell in love with the beach**.

She had her own famous Celebrate Life expression that she would yell out when she was feeling really good or happy about something like getting B-I-N-G-O or making a great toss in a Bocce match.

"Wee Pee Dee!"

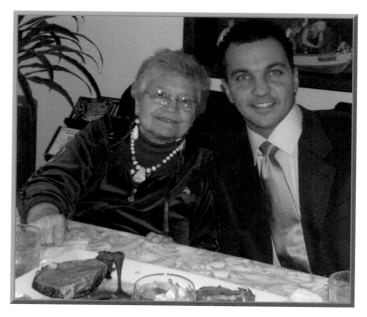

With Grandma Pedalino

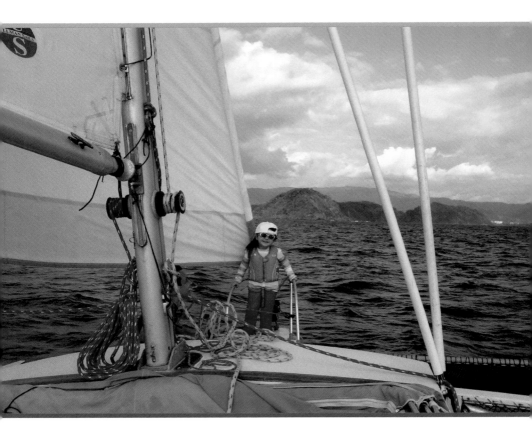

To this day, just reminiscing with my family about our days down the shore and Grandma Dora makes everyone smile with fondness and gratitude.

As someone who **can't stand people who don't *walk the walk,*** I'm proud to report that Isabella has already been to Costa Rica. *She makes the trip with me annually and she loves it.* It's **our little family tradition** that *she* gets to look forward to each year. This is my version of **passing on something good** to the next generation.

I'll happily die with nothing in the bank knowing that I gave her everything I had while I was here.

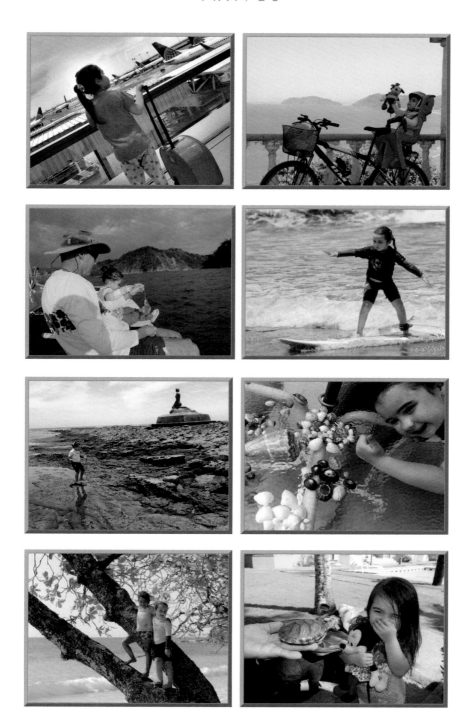

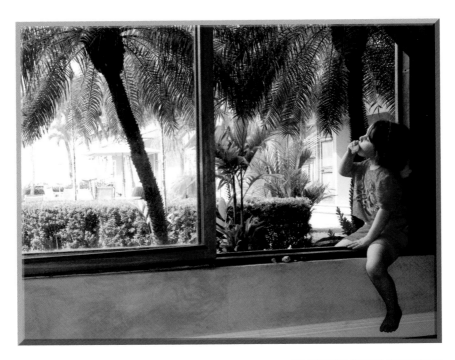

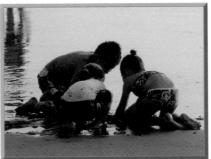

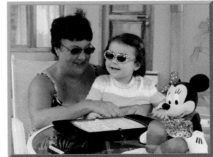

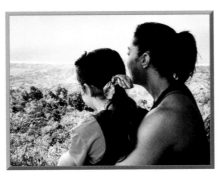

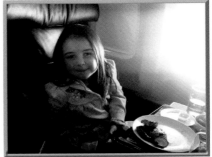

#CelebrateLife

1 Save up a little money, pick a destination, and book a flight. It's that simple. Not sure where to go? Determine your destination by narrowing down your personal preferences. *Snow, sun, surf, art, architecture, adventure, history, spiritual, loud, chill, cooking classes, etc.* You can even pick your favorite language. The world is waiting!

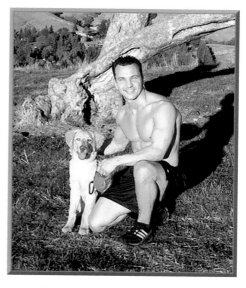

Trail running on Brioni Hill with "Buster" in California

If you're too nervous to travel without a personal recommendation, consult your VIPs. (see Chapter 2) They've probably seen some of the best destinations out there already and would be happy to suggest a few possibilities.

2   The friendlier you are, the less expensive it is. When cool friends come to town, offer to have them stay with you for a few days or at least be as gracious and helpful as possible during their trip. This way, when your schedule opens up and you can go on a little micro adventure, you can comfortably ask if they can assist you with *your* itinerary this time around. The worst that can happen is they say "no", the best that can happen is that they say "yes", and you can save yourself a large part of the traveling expense. Even better, you might have some fantastic friends, like Ron and Jill Michaels from Colorado or Dan and Darlene Ohrman from California, who are also outdoor enthusiasts, who will gladly open their doors, treat you like family, and be better tour guides than anyone you could have ever hired.

3   Create an account on *instagram* and follow some remarkable modern day explorers like *Jessica Stein* who will inspire you to travel abroad and remind you that "not all those who wander are lost."

4   If money is too tight, or some of life's challenges are making a one-day getaway the only logistically practical option right now, hop in the car and drive to the nearest ocean or lake. Other than pretending to be friends with someone you don't really care for, just to chill out at their pool for a few hours, this is probably your best option for finding a suitable local oasis.

*Just because you are in "oasis mode" for the day, it doesn't mean you should disregard reality and eat poorly for eighteen hours and wake up the next day feeling awful. Instead of eating at the snack shacks and fast food places that are usually located on site at most beach and lake properties, I recommend that you be self-sufficient with your sustenance instead. *It'll take about thirty minutes to shop for the groceries at your local food market, about thirty minutes to prepare the meals and snacks at your home, and will cost about $75 for two people ... but,* you'll be in control of the menu, the quality of selections, the size of the portions, and have everything at your fingertips so you won't impulsively go for those over-priced slices of pizza, greasy hot dogs, fried cheese sticks, or ice cream that they are conveniently selling twenty yards away. The bottom line is that you'll actually be saving money and eating better food from breakfast through dinner.

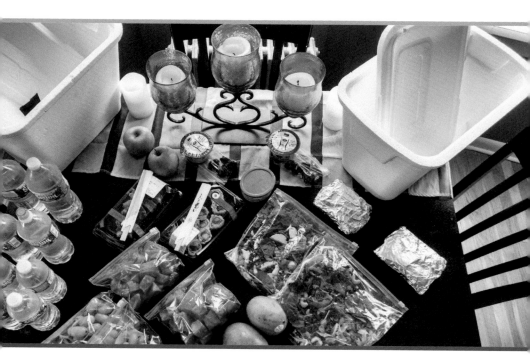

A full day's worth of healthy meals and snacks with portable refrigeration

Here is a sample menu for two:

	(8) Bottles of water.
	(2) Styrofoam coolers. Pack the water and some of the fruit in one cooler, put the remaining items in the other cooler.
	(2) 8 lb. bags of ice. *Pack ice in large zip lock bags to the keep the food, especially the wraps and sushi, dry from the moisture and water that the melting ice produces throughout the day.
1:30pm	Sushi and Mango.
4:00pm	Spring mix salad with grilled chicken, blue cheese, walnuts, cranberries, and balsamic dressing. *Pack dressing and walnuts separately so the salad and nuts do not lose their crunch.
4:30pm	Yogurt, prunes, and almonds.
7:30pm	Turkey, roast beef, Swiss cheese, red peppers, and hummus wraps.
8:00pm	Grapes.
Back up snack	Apples.
Don't forget	Dental floss. *You'll need it after the mango. Plastic spoons and forks for the salad and yogurt. Napkins.

Not pictured on page 73:

9:30am	Sweet Italian sausage, egg, and avocado burrito. Cup of green tea and a tablespoon of raw honey. Strawberries. *Since we have a 1.5 hour ride to the beach we do our workout first, have a protein shake, shop and prep for the outing, and then eat our breakfast on the way down the shore.

I pack my own green tea bag, raw honey, and 'to go' cup for the way home, too. I found a Dunkin Donuts that allows me to use its restroom and that will fill my cup with hot water before I start my journey back.

I bought the Dunkin Donuts' green tea and honey on my first trip but didn't care for it at all. No worries. I just bring my own each time now so it's exactly what I want.

Marcello's Message

Don't wait for someone to bring you flowers;
plant your own garden instead.

I always offer to pay for the hot water, but the young lady just smiles and fills up the cup. Although I'm not a fan of Dunkin Donuts and need to stay away from all their tantalizing baked goods, I am a fan of their Long Branch, New Jersey location. Kudos to the smiling and friendly counter attendant who usually works in the evening on weekends.

Cruising back home after a beautiful day at the beach with the top down and a delicious cup of tea in hand is nothing short of living it up for me. When I get to share moments like these with someone special or my family, the fulfillment factor goes up exponentially.

Remember, they don't put U-haul on your hearse. You can't take it with you.

Don't make your friends and family wait until your eulogy to talk about how much fun you've all been having.

Mae West nailed it when she said, *"You only live once ... but if you do it right, once is enough."*

CHAPTER 5

Make A Difference

"All that we are is the result of what we have thought: it is founded on thoughts, it is made up of our thoughts. If a person speaks or acts with an evil thought, pain follows him, as the wheel follows the foot of the ox that draws the wagon ... If a person speaks or acts with a pure thought, happiness follows him, like a shadow that never leaves him."

—THE DHAMMAPADA

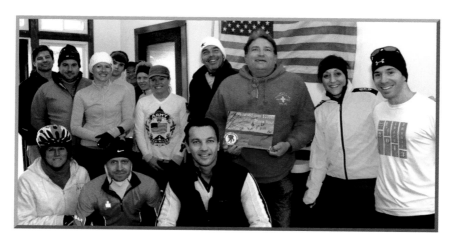

In Sparta, NJ for the Track Friday "Lake Mohawk Run & Ride" for Wounded Warriors

From top left: Todd Muth, Arturo Ruiz, Aleksandra Maz, Michael Contaxis, Ron Contaxis, Terri Contaxis, Lauren Huffman, Michael Walter, George Panzitta, Dr. Jill Garripoli, Eric Rubinson

Bottom left: Lisa Goldman Truesdale, Marek Bykuc, & Marcello Pedalino

If you are already taking good care of yourself, surrounding yourself with inspiring people, embracing the journey, doing what you love, AND traveling the world ... it's time to give back. *Actually, it's always a great time to give back.* In this chapter, you'll learn a few ways to have a lot of fun, make the world a better place, and make a big difference in someone's life all at the same time.

I'm a sucker for a feel-good movie so seeing the underdog win, watching the unlikely boy getting the girl of his dreams, or giving someone who needs a second chance the tools to make things right—is even more magical when it happens in real life.

And, if you believe in Karma or agree with the notion that "what goes around comes around," it's one of those rare win-win situations where everyone *actually* wins without any fine print or any shady email-from-Nigeria type of shenanigans.

Marcello's Message

If you want to feel good about yourself, be good to other people.

I've always had a soft spot in my heart for veterans. Not only because of how much I value the independence and freedom they've given to me to Celebrate Life daily, but because they've got more guts and bravery than I'll ever have. They are a special breed of human beings that deserve every ounce of respect one can muster—and not just on a few 'holidays' each year, but *every* day.

Recently, my hilariously-witty friend and superhero-like runner, Eric Rubinson, (*who ran fifty marathons—one in every state*) inspired me to contribute to his fundraiser.

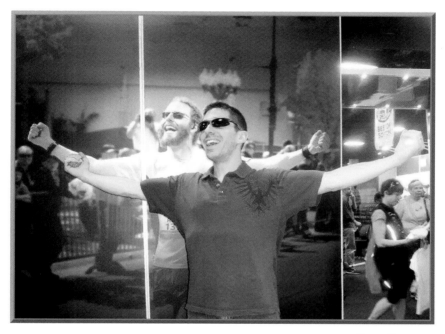

Eric Rubenson

He created "Track Friday" to raise money for victims of Hurricane Sandy and to encourage all do-gooders to help out any cause they see fit, *while getting fit* at the same time. **Eric's movement is based on getting off your butt the day after Thanksgiving (Black Friday) to get some much needed post-gluttonous exercise and raise money for your favorite charity *instead* of getting up at the crack of dawn just to act like a Neanderthal and knock someone over at Walmart to save $28 on another flat screen TV that you *don't* need for your house.**

I organized a nine mile run and bike ride around my new neighborhood, Lake Mohwak, in Sparta NJ, and raised a nice chunk of change for the Wounded Warrior Project with the help of some dear friends, including Eric, who made the trip up to join me. **No doubt, it was one of the most rewarding days of my life.** Having a blast, solidifying friendships, and getting a great workout all while paying it forward was a bonus. A **check can't even begin to show the thanks and appreciation I have for all the warriors who nearly sacrificed it all—like some**, but it's *something.*

Marcello's Message

Sometimes doing whatever you can within your means and ability to help out is much better than doing nothing at all.

#CelebrateLife

1 Whether it's a physical RAK (Random Act of Kindness) or a monetary donation to a buddy's charity, **there's no excuse not to give something back and make a nice deposit in the bank of goodwill.** Not sure where to start? Go outside and pick up some trash that's on an elderly neighbor's lawn. Then, go find out who threw it there and go throw it back on *their* lawn. *Just kidding.*

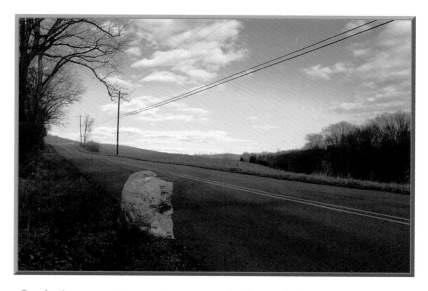

Don't forget a heavy duty pair of gloves before you go out and "Give a Hoot" (so you don't cut yourself on a broken bottle and get 6 stitches in your hand)

2 If you have old clothes, or anything you haven't worn in over a year or doesn't fit you anymore, (see Chapter 1) donate them immediately. You'll reclaim some space in the closet and most likely help out someone who actually needs a decent outfit for a job interview.

There are some great organizations out there, like the Renovation House here in NJ. They help substance abusers turn their lives around with a one year commitment that requires graduating from a recovery and educational program. It has an eighty percent success rate. After making some healthier nutrition choices over the past few years and dropping a size, that's where a bunch of my suits went.

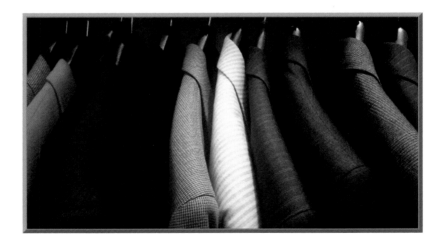

3 Volunteer for Habitat for Humanity like my dad does. Don't worry if you can't frame a house or install the electrical and plumbing by yourself, neither can my dad. They've got experienced folks on site to handle all the Bob Villa stuff.

What you can do is just about everything else because HFH will put you with a group of great people whose various levels of experience and abilities create a well-rounded and productive team. You'll make a big difference for a family who is in need of disaster relief and also make some wonderful new friends. If you are not retired like my dad, and you don't have the time to donate your physical labor, you can also donate materials or make a financial donation instead. There's always a way to help.

4   Donate some of your airline miles to a charity or a cause that's having a fundraiser.

5   Find and follow someone like my friend Ron Michaels on social media. He's always running, biking, or hiking up scenic mountains for a great cause. Support him with a financial donation or take a trip out to Colorado and join him on an upcoming adventure. Reaching the summit of Mt. Elbert to raise money for the Larimer Humane Society was an incredible experience. (see cover photo for Chapter 4)

6   Mentor someone. If you are really good at something and see someone with potential, reach out to them and offer a little guidance. If they are receptive and you get the warm fuzzies for paying it forward, it's all good. When a person knows that someone else believes in them and is on their side, it makes a world of difference in their self-confidence.

I think comedic filmmaker and producer Judd Apatow has a great take on mentorship.

"One reason I was able to build a career is because of the advice I got from people ... When I had the ability to help others, it felt like the natural thing to do. I do that because people like Gary Shandling were kind to me when I was figuring out how to be a writer and a comedian."

7　If you can type and are using any social media platform, write a blog or post about your favorite cause or organization to help promote their message.

8　If you've got decent hand writing, volunteer to write little thank you notes to donors from your favorite cause or organization.

9　Do you have a friend who is fighting cancer or some other horrible disease? Volunteer to babysit their kids, take their dog for a walk, or help tidy up their house. You can also just listen. Sometimes, they just want to share their raw thoughts or simply take comfort in your company without having to say anything at all.

10　While writing this book, my friend's son, Christopher D'Amico Jr., left this world too soon. His parents rallied and started a national campaign called Kindness for Christopher. "On the 24th day of every month, do at least one random act of kindness for someone. It doesn't have to be monetary. It could be as simple as looking at somebody and telling them they look nice that day or holding the door open for somebody. Just go out of your way to make someone's life a little easier. Maybe buy a cup of coffee for somebody. Paying it forward, essentially."

CHAPTER 6

Let It Go

"Holding onto anger is like grasping a hot coal with the intent of throwing it at someone else; you are the one who gets burned."

— Buddha

If you're a parent, grandparent, aunt, uncle, or a glutton for pop culture one hit wonders, "Let It Go" are three words that either made you smile wide and start singing or roll your eyes just now. In this chapter, you'll learn how this mantra transcends a world famous animated movie. Recognizing what "It" is and **letting "It" go is paramount if you want to truly Celebrate Life. If you don't** *Let It Go,* **you'll be trapped in the wrath of the past or the joy-stealing web of agonizing too much over what the future** *might* **bring.**

So maybe you got screwed over, jerked around, kicked below the belt, stepped on, knocked down, disrespected, or treated like a second class citizen and therefore held a grudge bigger than Mt. Everest.

Or, maybe you hit the jackpot like me and had to deal with all seven lovely categories at once.

Well, let me offer you a little piece of unsolicited advice that is **much easier said than done** … *Let It Go.*

The ability to let it go and *forgive* is vital.

However, to be **crystal clear,** I'm not suggesting that you *forget* what happened. You don't want to make the same mistake twice. **If the guilty parties did it once, they'll likely do it again if given the opportunity.**

What I *am* saying is, **don't dwell on the part that hurts so much.** Instead, **focus on and draw strength from the fact that you are** *Unbroken* and just like my mom said, "*the sun will shine again.*"

If you haven't seen the movie **Unbroken** *yet, the story of World War II Veteran* **Louie Zamperini** *who survived forty seven days* at sea and a series of hellish prisoner of war camps, put it on your 'must see' list. It's an amazing true story of **survival, resilience, and redemption.**

Marcello's Message

The reality is, sometimes there is no silver lining, such as in the case of a tragedy or when you lose a loved one.

However, in most cases, there is indeed a sense of new hope that rises from the ashes that would never have been possible without the inferno you endured.

And in *some* cases, your situation can actually have the happily-ever-after ending in the spirit of the 6 Million Dollar Man. **You'll not only triumph, you'll be reincarnated as a stronger, smarter, happier, and ultimately more fulfilled version of your previous self.**

I don't recommend taking **this particular route to discover fulfillment** if you can avoid it.

It's a doozy.

It hurts.

And it will push you right *over* the edge if you don't **have a great support system**. *I was fortunate to have one.*

However, like Frank Zamperini told his brother Louie when he was growing up, *"If you can take it, you can make it."*

I promised myself, for my daughter's sake, that I would never publicly speak ill about a few individuals and events that took place in the past.

Yes, my tongue is bloody from how many times I've had to bite it.

Instead, the **focus** would be on **living in the present** and surrounding Isabella and our home with as much **love, positive energy**, guidance, and **opportunities to thrive** as humanly possible.

A verbal gem from my awesome yoga instructor, Lisa Franey, has come in handy on more than one **"Let It Go"** occasion and is worth mentioning here ...

"Pain is inevitable, suffering is optional."

Done and done.

Gone.

#CelebrateLife

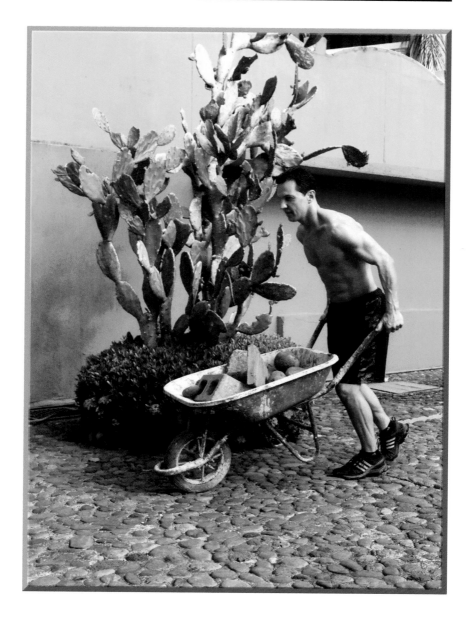

1 They say running is the cheapest form of therapy. I'd have to agree. (see Chapter 1) Bad knees ... can't run? Walk instead. Start by walking around your block and increase the distance as you get stronger. Can't walk? Hop on your bike. No bike? Buy a cheap one and start pedaling.
Start by riding around your block and increase the distance as you get stronger. Never learned how to ride a bike? Get in a pool, lake, or ocean and start swimming. *Enough* with the excuses. Take a cue from *Mike Connor*, a man who broke ninety percent of the bones in his body after a ghastly thirty foot fall. His motto is, "If you can move, you can exercise."

You can't let anything go without an outlet for your stress and unwelcomed negative mojo from VDPs. (see Chapter 2)

Buy a good pair of sneakers, a cheap pair of boxing gloves, and go join a gym, YMCA, or any place that has a heavy bag that you can punch as hard as you can for as long as it takes to release the tension.

If all else fails, go outside and create your own exercise program with stuff you already have. Put some rocks in a wheelbarrow and start walking. (see the previous page) *A huge tropical cactus bush is not necessary.*

What if you're broke and have no money to join a gym or a YMCA? What if you work from home, are a single parent, and the nearest workout facility is thirty minutes away? **No worries.** Do the same thing that you would do if you were traveling for business or pleasure and didn't have any fancy equipment to work with. **Use your body weight and go old school.**

Here's a sample of one of my old school
body weight workouts:

1 minute of jumping rope.

*A jump rope fits easily in any carry-on suitcase
with your sneakers.

25 pushups.

25 sit ups.

25 jumping jacks.

Walk or run a lap around the hotel. Bad weather?
Try ten flights of stairs. **No excuses.**

Repeat this set twice more or until you do at least a thirty
minute workout or until you have to get into the shower
to start your day.

*If you can a find a pullup bar or some type of ledge
that will allow you to do pull-ups or chin-ups, go for it.
I found these to be one of the best body weight
exercises out there.

2   If you don't get the same tension relief and reboot benefits from fitness that I do, no worries. Try writing (a little cathartic book like this) or even photography. Both are wonderful outlets for creativity and excellent ways to productively express your internal feelings. I actually love combining the hobbies and creating memes like you find on Pinterest by mashing up noteworthy quotes with some of my photos. Climbing up Red Rock mountain in Las Vegas with my awesome friend, Brian Snyder, was a really enjoyable experience when it happened but creating a meme helped us capture the therapeutic nature and long-term benefits of that magnificent day forever. (See the next page)

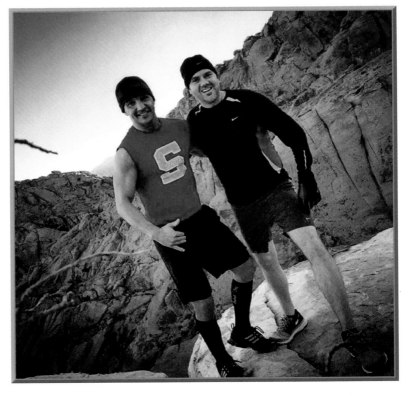

With Brian Snyder in Las Vegas

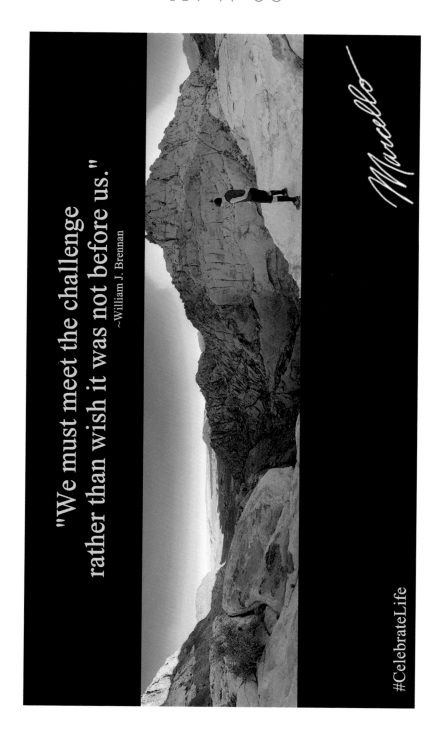

"We must meet the challenge
rather than wish it was not before us."
~William J. Brennan

Marcello

#CelebrateLife

Marcello's Message

If you keep your eyes, ears, and mind open,
you can find inspiration everywhere.

Here are a few more samples of the motivational memes
that I enjoy creating. Taking the photograph, in and of itself,
reduces stress and gets my creative juices flowing.
Combining it with some wisdom makes for a fun hobby and
a wonderful way to help *let things go* when needed.

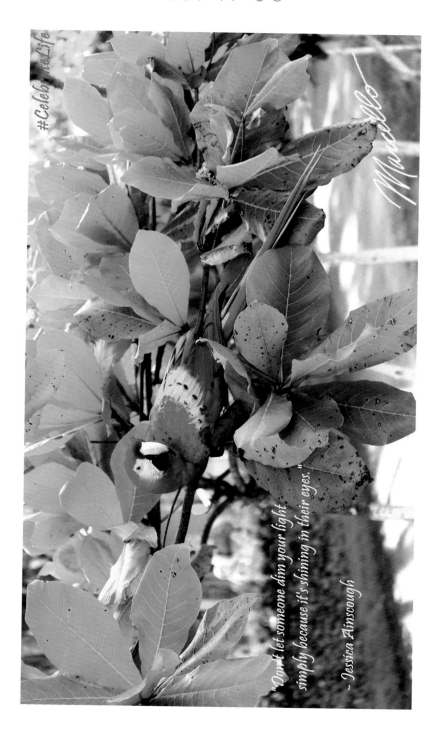

#Celebrate_Life

Marcello

"Don't let someone dim your light simply because it's shining in their eyes."

~ Jessica Ainscough

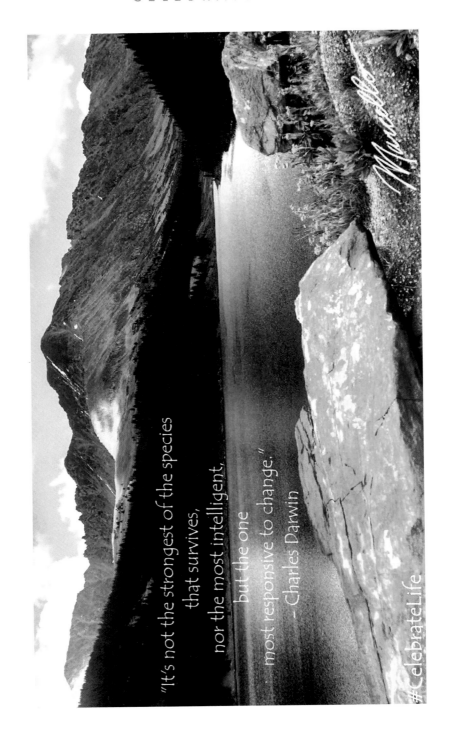

"It's not the strongest of the species
that survives,
nor the most intelligent,
but the one
most responsive to change."
– Charles Darwin

#CelebrateLife

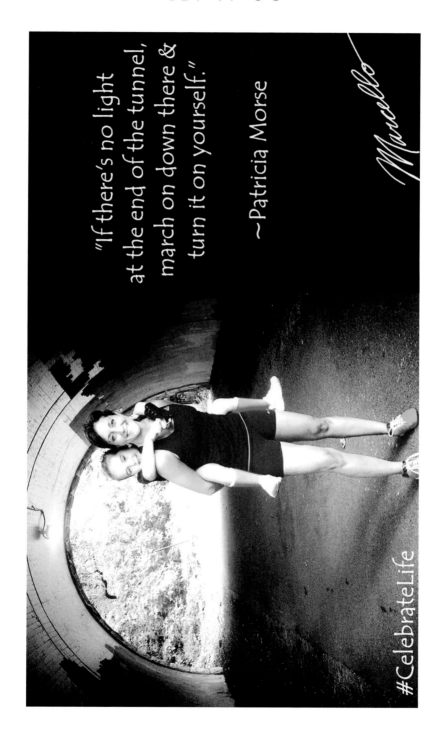

"If there's no light at the end of the tunnel, march on down there & turn it on yourself."

~Patricia Morse

Marcello

#CelebrateLife

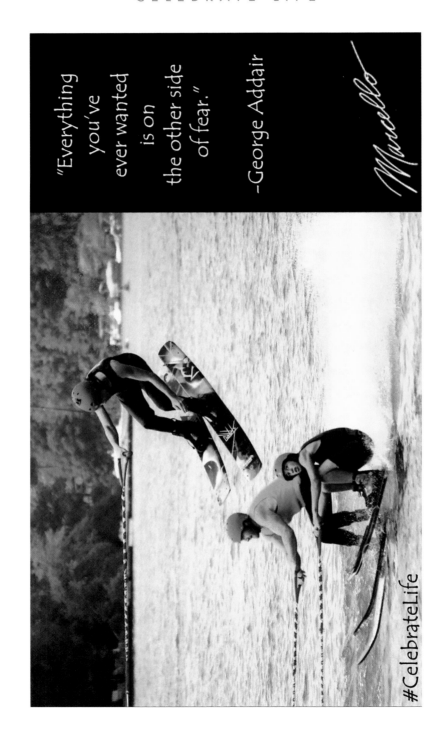

"Everything
you've
ever wanted
is on
the other side
of fear."

–George Addair

Marcello

#CelebrateLife

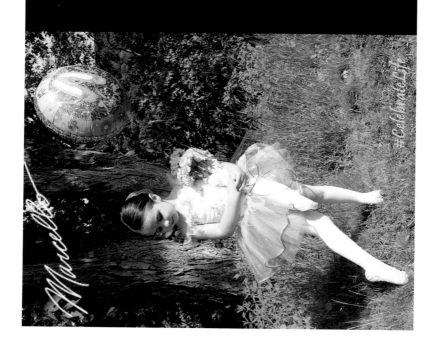

"Beauty might be a gift
to our souls from the heavens.

Luxury, purchased.

But suddenly she understood,
there was strength in elegance."

~Lynn Sheene

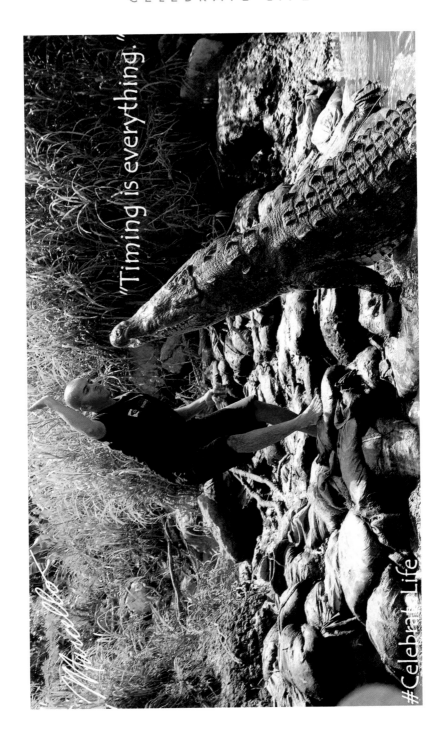

"Timing is everything."

#CelebrateLife

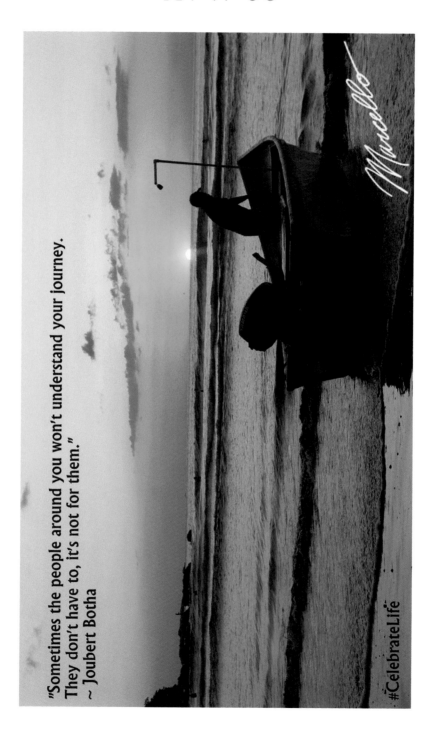

"Sometimes the people around you won't understand your journey. They don't have to, it's not for them."
~ Joubert Botha

#CelebrateLife

Marcello

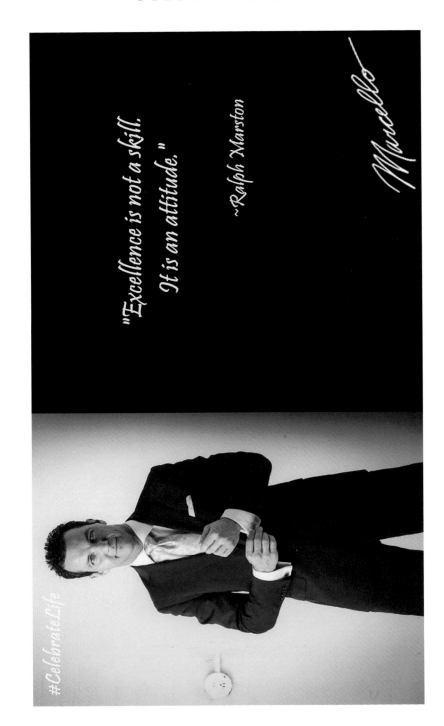

"Excellence is not a skill.
It is an attitude."

~Ralph Marston

Marcello

#CelebrateLife

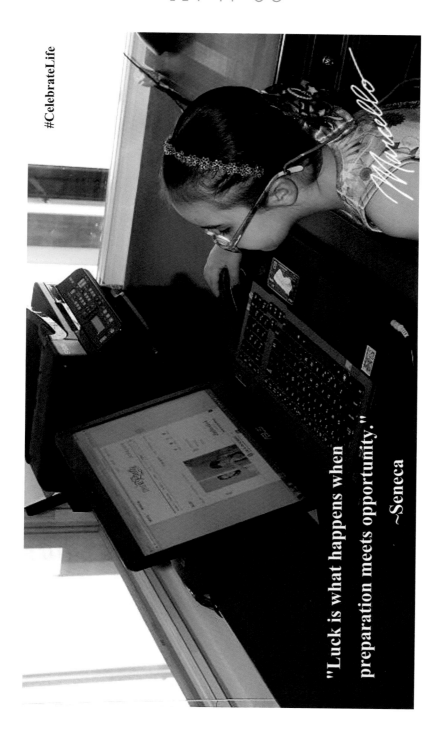

#CelebrateLife

"Luck is what happens when preparation meets opportunity."

~Seneca

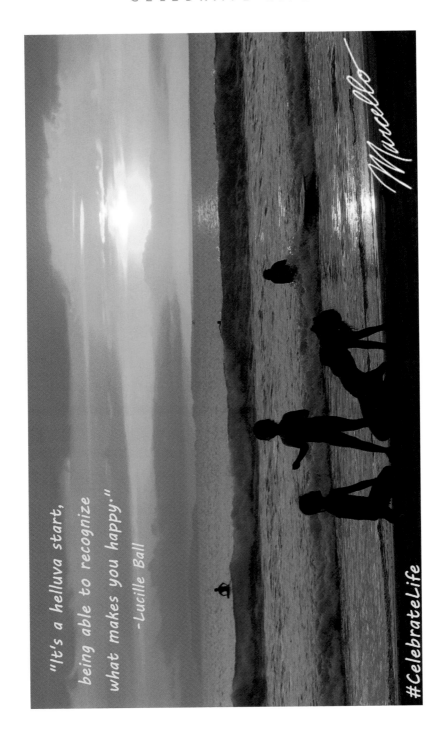

"It's a helluva start, being able to recognize what makes you happy."

—Lucille Ball

Marcello

#CelebrateLife

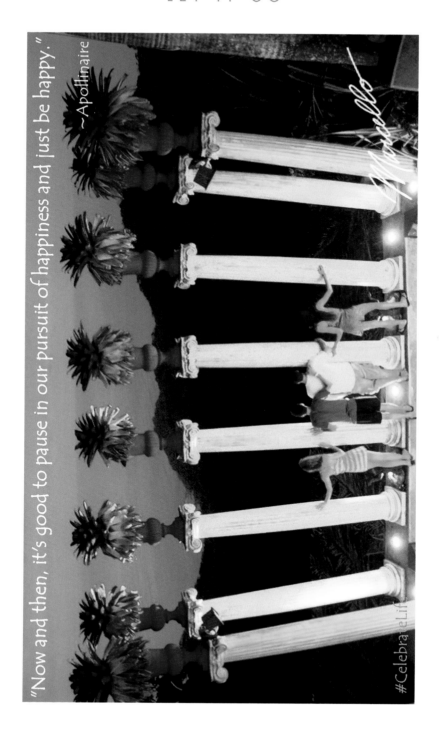

"Now and then, it's good to pause in our pursuit of happiness and just be happy."
~Apollinaire

Marcello

#CelebrateLife

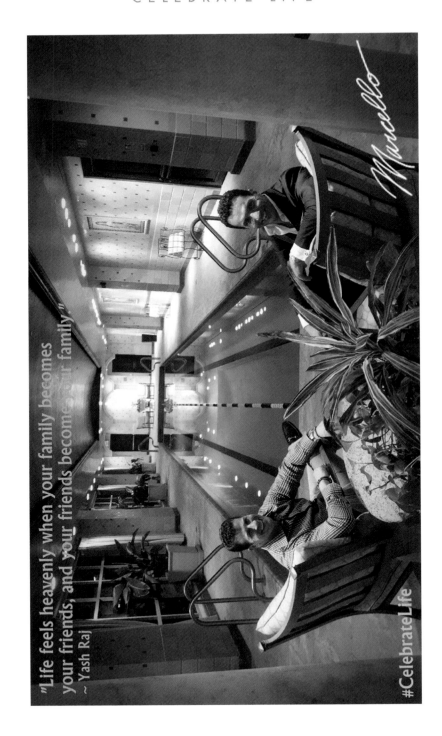

"Life feels heavenly when your family becomes your friends, and your friends become your family."
~ Yash Raj

#CelebrateLife

Marcello

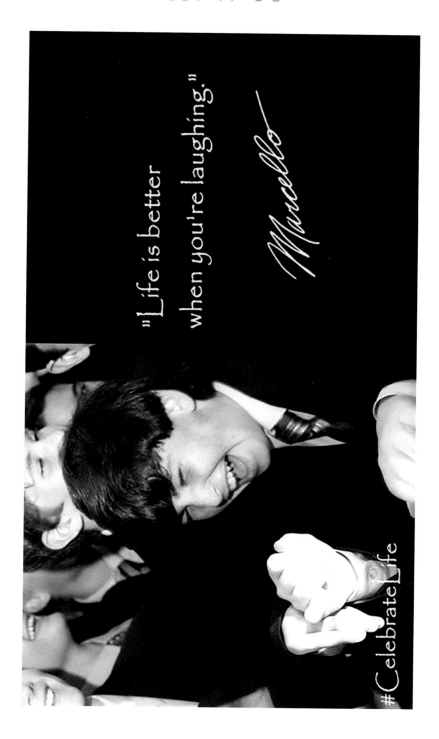

"Life is better when you're laughing."

Marcello

#CelebrateLife

"The quality of a father
can be seen
in the goals, dreams, and aspirations
he sets not only for himself,
but for his family."

~ Reed Markham

I love you Dad.

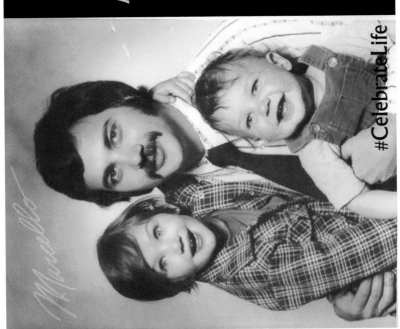

#CelebrateLife

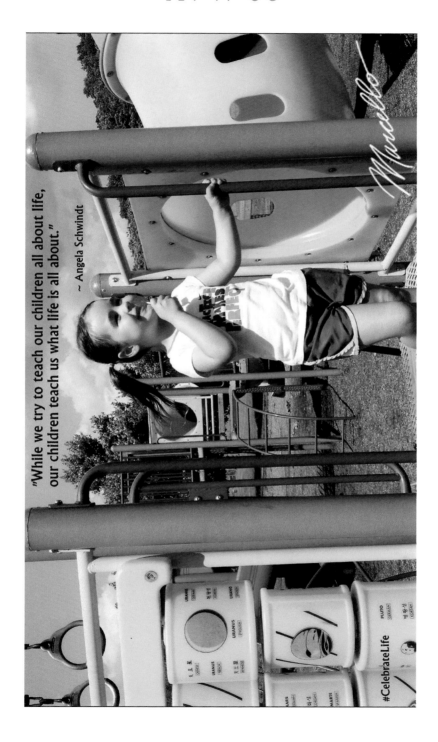

"While we try to teach our children all about life,
our children teach us what life is all about."

~ Angela Schwindt

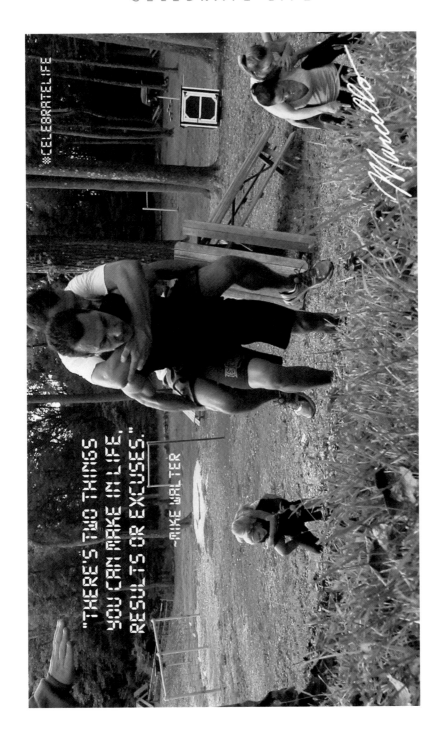

If you'd like to make your own memes, all you need is:

- a camera or mobile device to take the picture.
- ten minutes on google to find a great quote.
- access to a basic site like MemeMaker.net or a program like Photoshop.

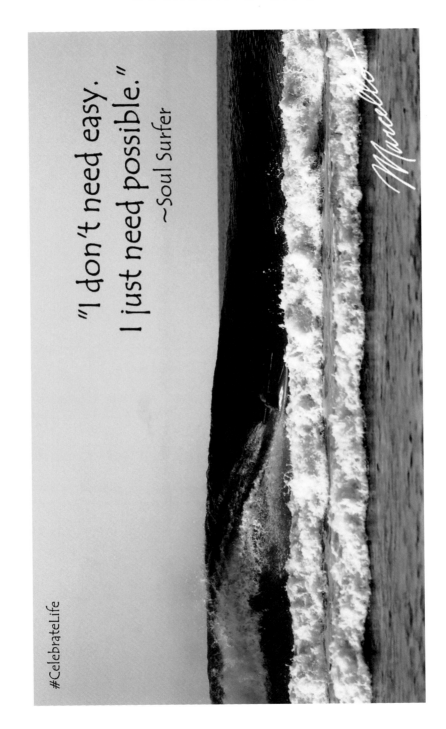

"I don't need easy.
I just need possible."
~Soul Surfer

Marcello

#CelebrateLife

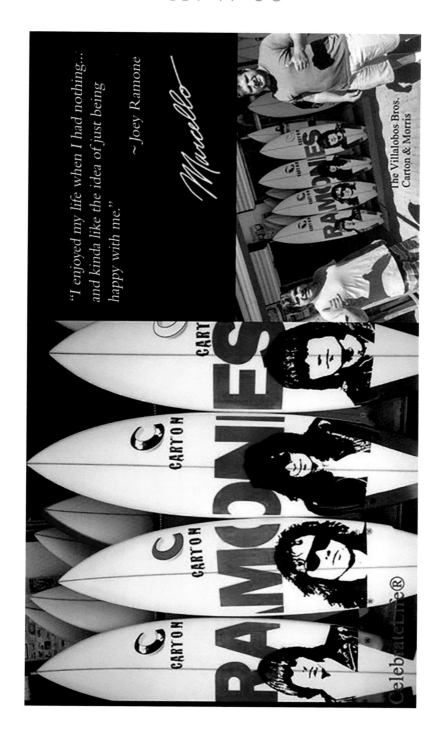

"I enjoyed my life when I had nothing... and kinda like the idea of just being happy with me."

~ Joey Ramone

Marcello

The Villalobos Bros.
Carton & Morris

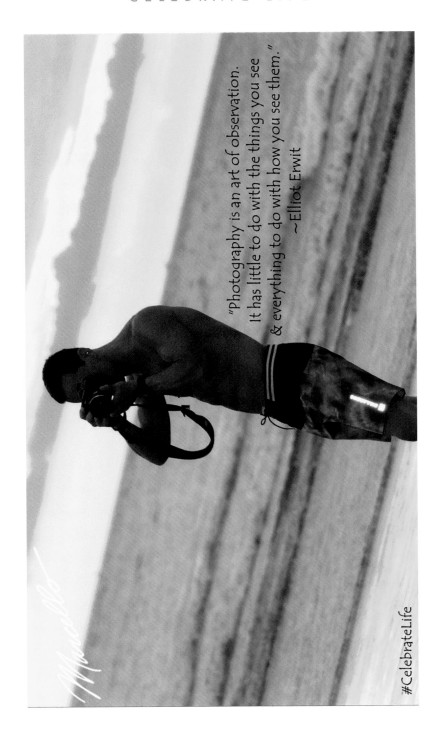

"Photography is an art of observation.
It has little to do with the things you see
& everything to do with how you see them."
~Elliot Erwit

#CelebrateLife

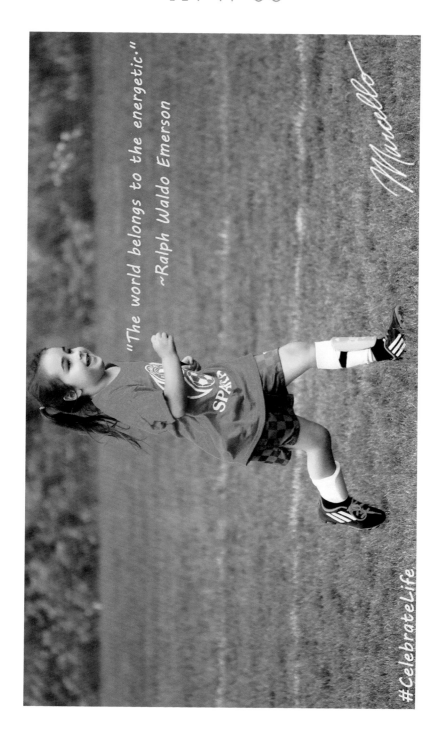

"The world belongs to the energetic."
~Ralph Waldo Emerson

Marcello

#CelebrateLife.

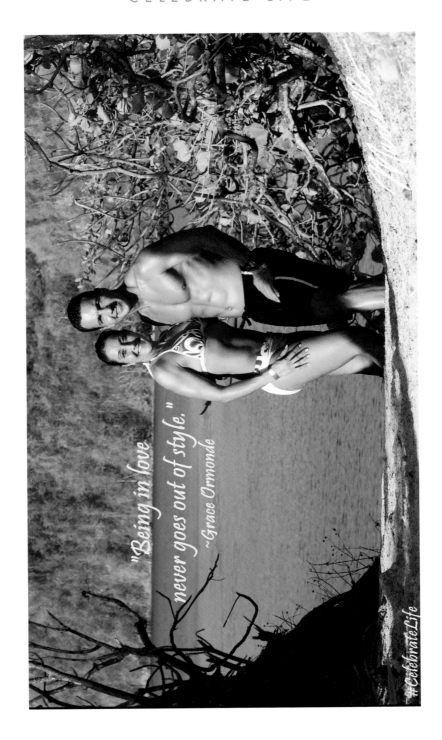

"Being in love
never goes out of style."
~Grace Ormonde

#CelebrateLife

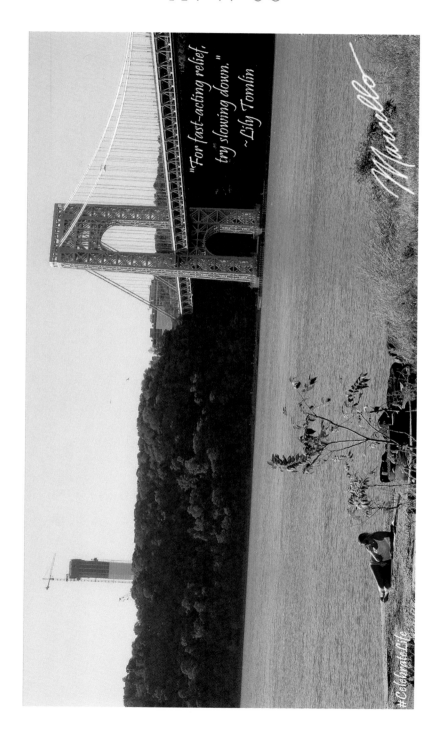

"For fast-acting relief, try slowing down." ~Lily Tomlin

Marcello

#CelebrateLife

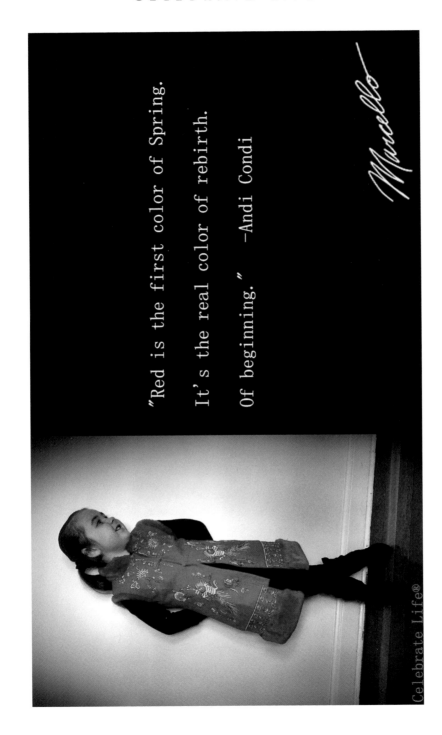

"Red is the first color of Spring.

It's the real color of rebirth.

Of beginning." —Andi Condi

Marcello

Celebrate Life®

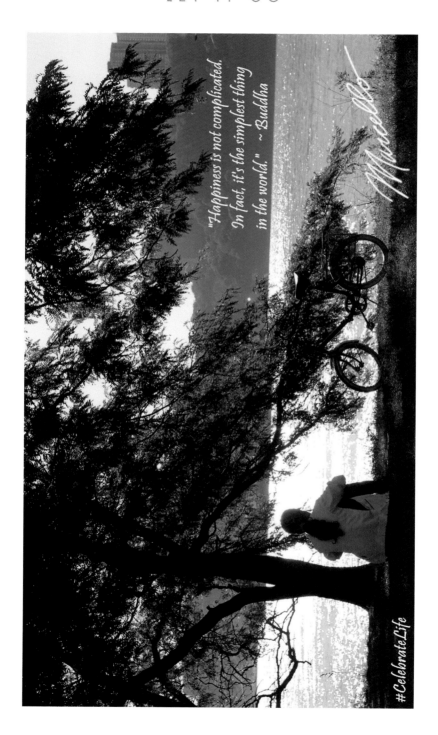

"Happiness is not complicated. In fact, it's the simplest thing in the world." ~ Buddha

Marcello

#CelebrateLife

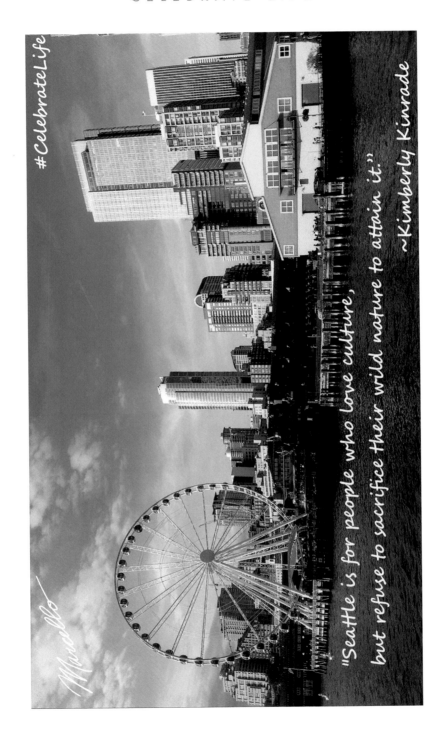

#CelebrateLife

"Seattle is for people who love culture, but refuse to sacrifice their wild nature to attain it."

~Kimberly Kinrade

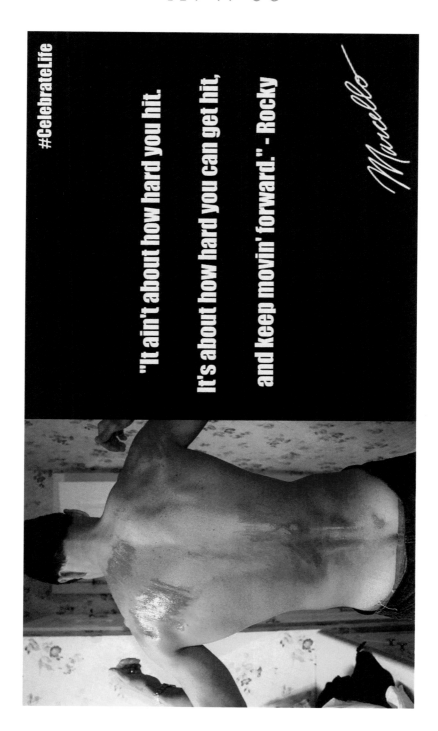

#CelebrateLife

"It ain't about how hard you hit.

It's about how hard you can get hit,

and keep movin' forward." - Rocky

Marcello

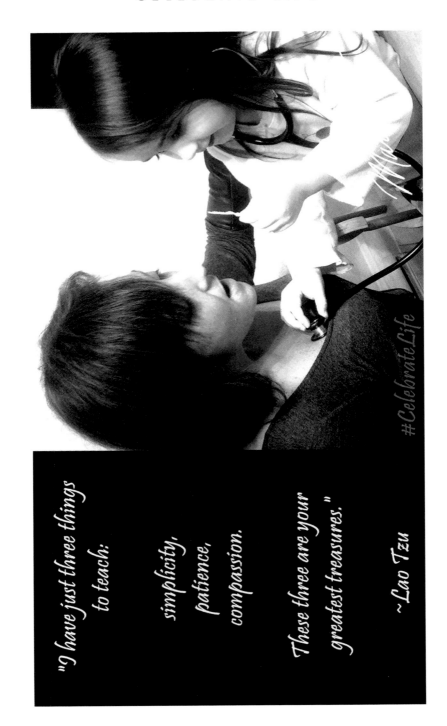

"I have just three things to teach:

simplicity,
patience,
compassion.

These three are your greatest treasures."

~Lao Tzu

#CelebrateLife

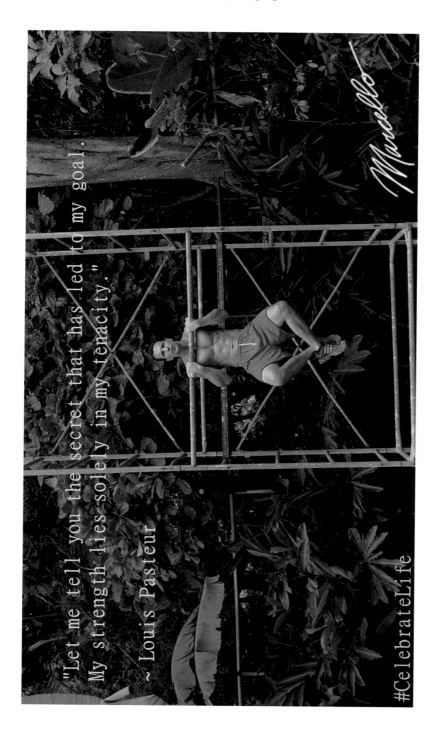

"Let me tell you the secret that has led to my goal. My strength lies solely in my tenacity."

~ Louis Pasteur

#CelebrateLife

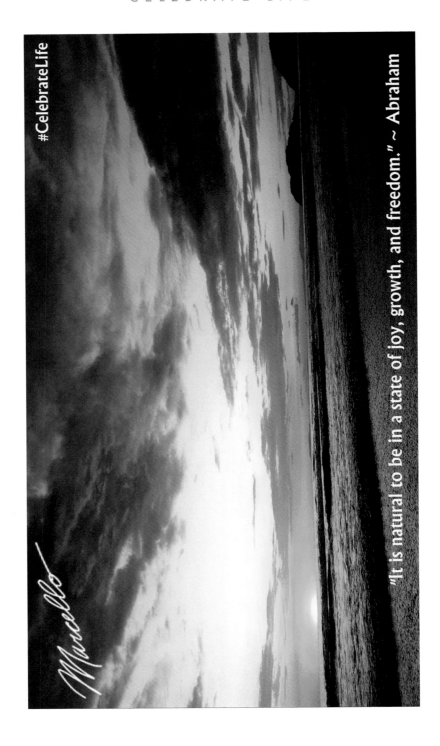

#CelebrateLife

Marcello

"It is natural to be in a state of joy, growth, and freedom." ~ Abraham

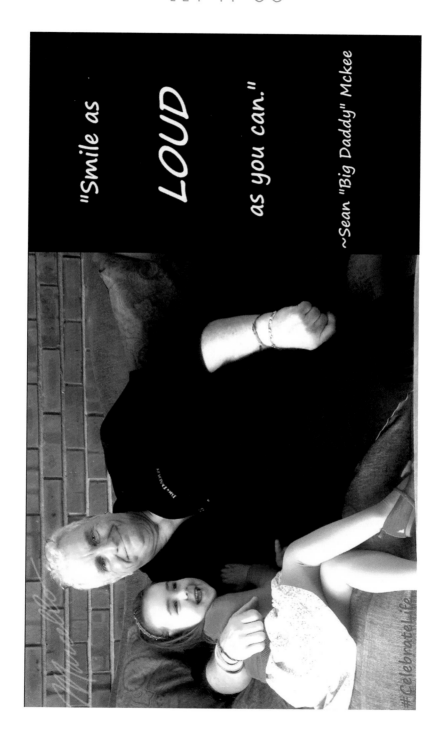

"Smile as *LOUD* as you can."

~Sean "Big Daddy" Mckee

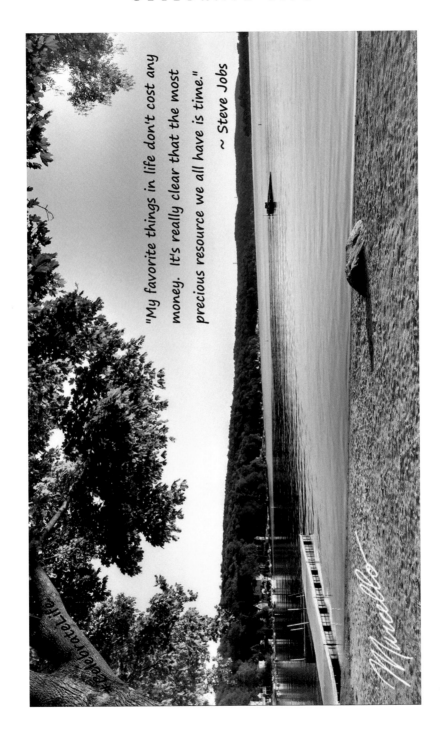

"My favorite things in life don't cost any money. It's really clear that the most precious resource we all have is time."

~ Steve Jobs

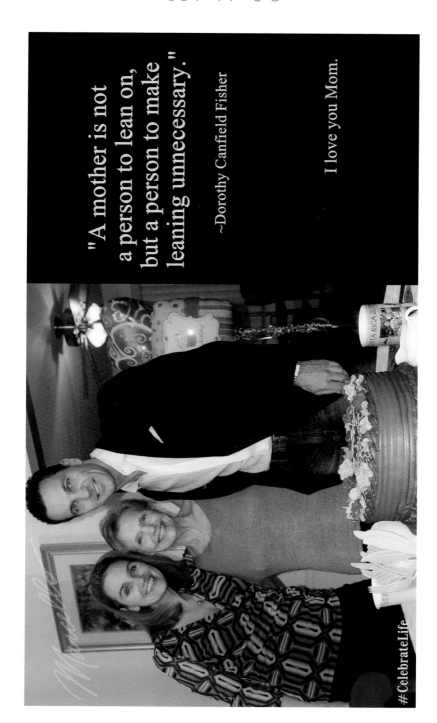

"A mother is not a person to lean on, but a person to make leaning unnecessary."

~Dorothy Canfield Fisher

I love you Mom.

#CelebrateLife

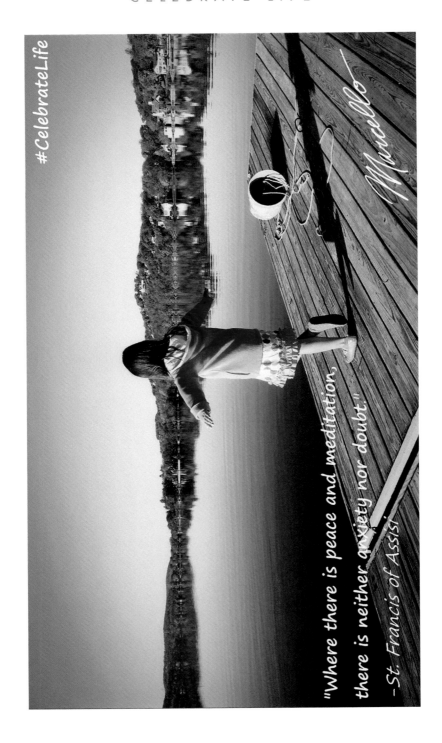

#CelebrateLife

"Where there is peace and meditation, there is neither anxiety nor doubt."
—St. Francis of Assisi

Marcello

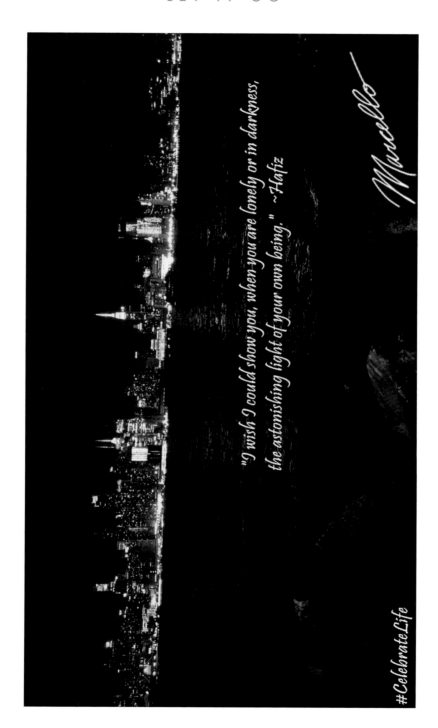

"I wish I could show you, when you are lonely or in darkness, the astonishing light of your own being." ~Hafiz

Marcello

#CelebrateLife

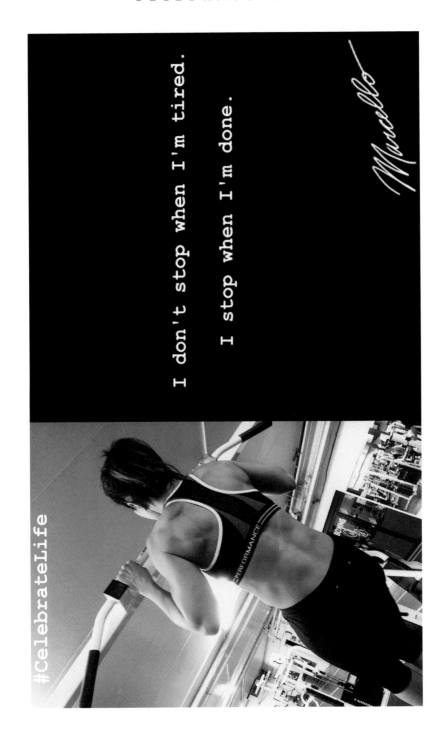

I don't stop when I'm tired.

I stop when I'm done.

Marcello

#CelebrateLife

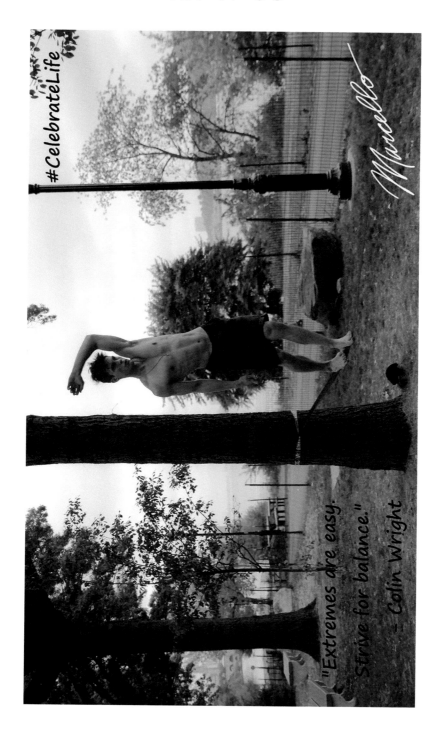

#CelebrateLife

Marcello

"Extremes are easy.
Strive for balance."
- Colin Wright

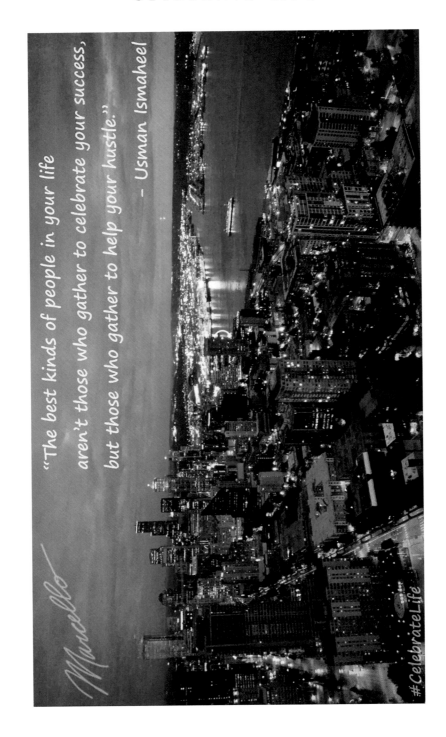

"The best kinds of people in your life aren't those who gather to celebrate your success, but those who gather to help your hustle."

– Usman Ismaheel

Marcello

#CelebrateLife

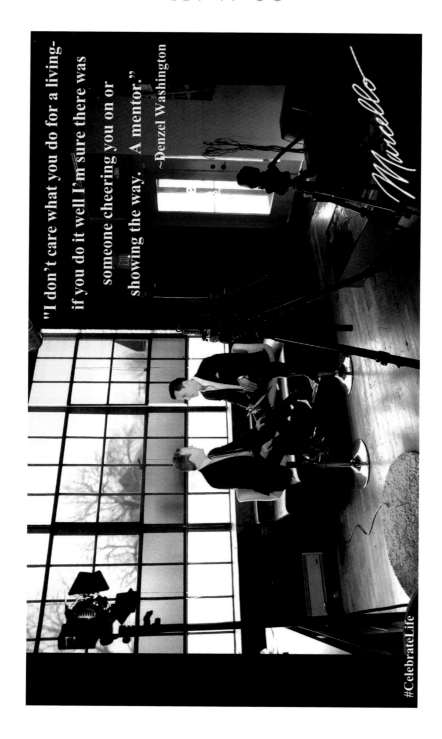

"I don't care what you do for a living- if you do it well I'm sure there was someone cheering you on or showing the way. A mentor."
~Denzel Washington

Marcello

#CelebrateLife

133

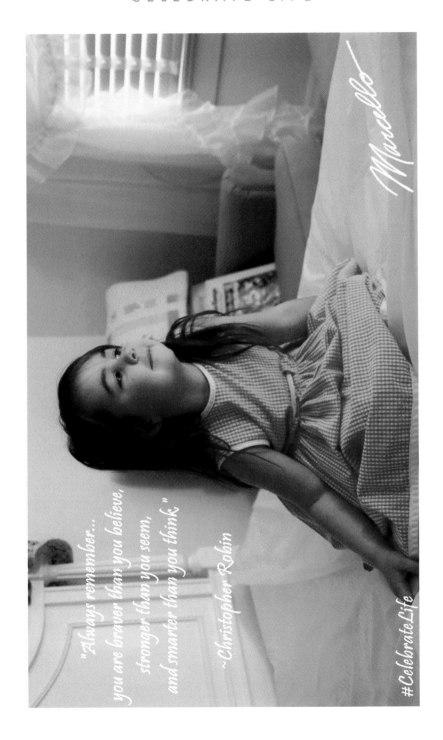

Marcello

*"Always remember...
you are braver than you believe,
stronger than you seem,
and smarter than you think."
~Christopher Robin*

#CelebrateLife

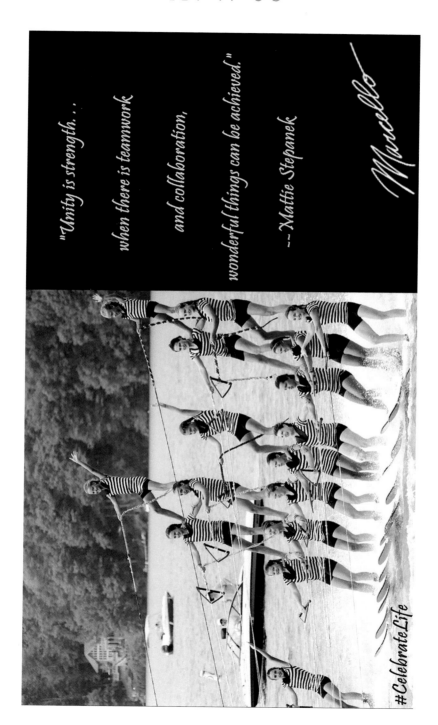

"Unity is strength. . . when there is teamwork and collaboration, wonderful things can be achieved."

~ Mattie Stepanek

Marcello

#CelebrateLife

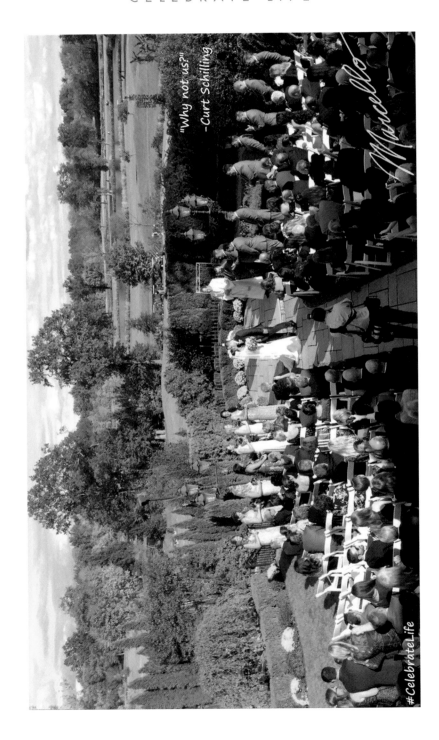

"Why not us?"
–Curt Schilling

Marcello

#CelebrateLife

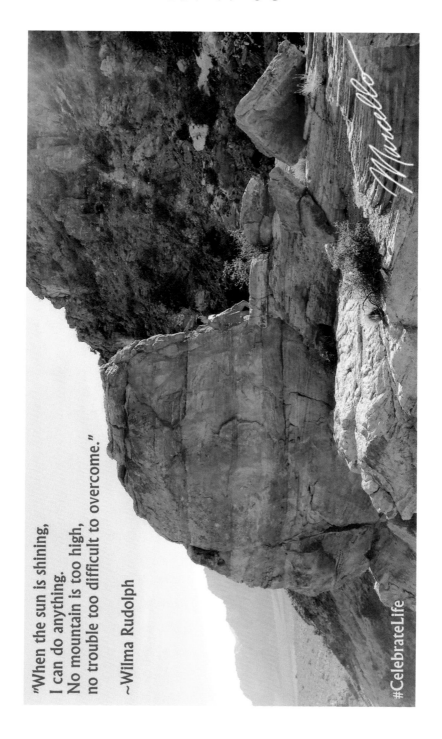

"When the sun is shining,
I can do anything.
No mountain is too high,
no trouble too difficult to overcome."

~Wilma Rudolph

#CelebrateLife

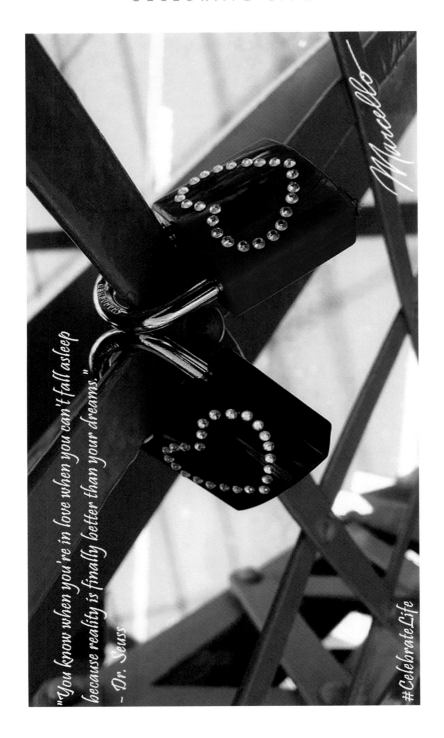

"You know when you're in love when you can't fall asleep because reality is finally better than your dreams."
– Dr. Seuss

Marcello

#CelebrateLife

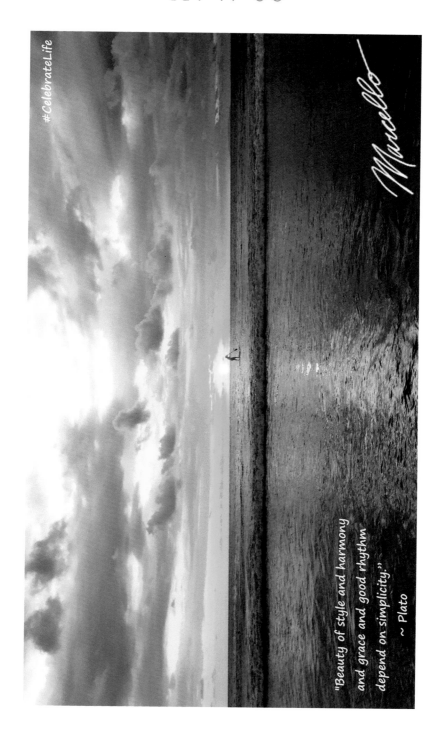

#CelebrateLife

"Beauty of style and harmony
and grace and good rhythm
depend on simplicity."
~ Plato

Marcello

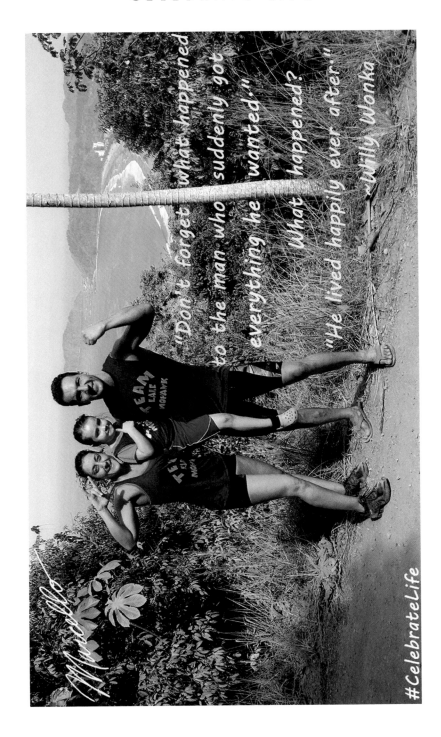

"Don't forget what happened to the man who suddenly got everything he wanted."

What happened?

"He lived happily ever after." —Willy Wonka

#CelebrateLife

Before you know it, your head will be clearer. You'll be able to rid yourself of all the poisonous distractions and instead **refocus on your life's priorities.**

3 Then, take a vacation or sabbatical that rejuvenates your mind, body, and spirit. (see Chapter 5) If done correctly and responsibly, you'll return in better shape than when you left and **a consistent wellness** program will soon become a non-negotiable addition to your everyday schedule.

CHAPTER

Evolve

7

"Twenty years from now you will be more disappointed by the things that you didn't do than by the ones you did do."

—MARK TWAIN

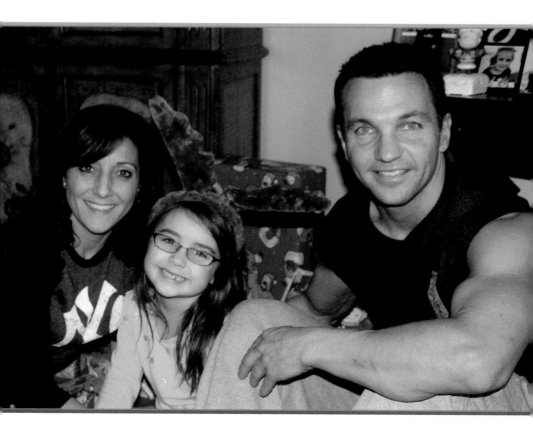

After you've let it go, gotten your wellness routine on point, found some more inspiring people, made a difference in someone else's life, discovered your passion, *AND* taken a rejuvenating excursion somewhere ... stop for a second and take a breather because you probably just had the best year of your life!

Marcello's Message

After survival, it's time to advance, rebuild, and refine.

Like most things in life, *if you've done it before, you can do it again.*

And if you can do it again, you can do it better.

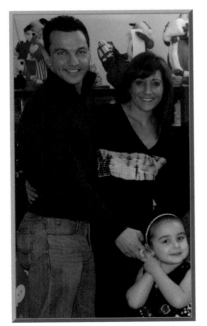

You've endured and conquered.

Sit for a moment and soak it all in. *Think Andy Dufrane in Shawshank when he made it out of the raw sewage pipe.*

I'm the first one to recognize the validity of the old saying, "If it ain't broke, don't fix it," but I'm also a strong proponent of the notion that you should "**stay humble *and* stay hungry.** " There are way too many hills you'll need to climb up in this world. **Coasting for the rest of your life *is*** *not and will never be* an option. **Forward motion and progress** via enhanced **open-mindedness,** and therefore better decision making skills, will always be essential to continuing the pursuit of **"enough"** and the enjoyment of **a fulfilling existence**.

Dave Ramsey, a **brilliant financial advisor and radio host** said something on his radio show that **changed my life forever.** A guy called in who needed to sell his house, but was only getting less than stellar offers because it was a buyer's market. As usual, Dave gave him some **sound advice** for his particular situation—as well as for a lot of folks who sometimes

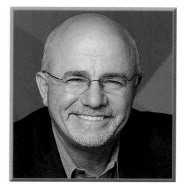

Dave Ramsey

have a tough time *letting it go.* (see Chapter 6) Dave got the listener to stop dead in his tracks when he offered up the words, **"to heck with the cheese, get out of the trap."**

That **sage counsel** has stuck with me ever since and helped me favor ***pragmatism over emotion*** on several challenging and otherwise conundrum-y occasions.

What's getting in the way of your personal evolution?

It took me a few years to figure that out, and **overcome the obstacles**.

#CelebrateLife

The funny thing about obtaining "enough," in the traditional sense of the word, is the humbling realization that you might actually need to get rid of some things to do it. *I think the fancy word for this is 'counterintuitive.'*

Sometimes taking a cautious *and terrifying* step backward is necessary in order to eventually gain momentum once again, and then thrust in the right direction with brazen fervor and resolve.

This is when the support of your friends and family is paramount.

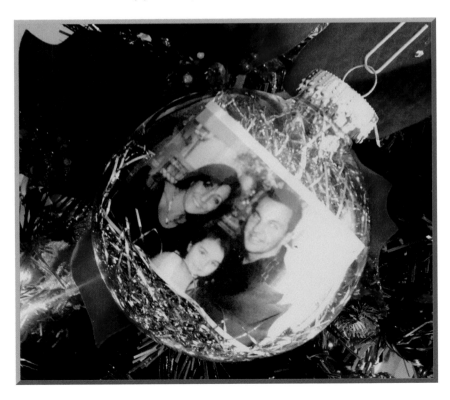

Marcello's Message

As much as you may not like asking for help, there is a time to put your ego aside and cash in a karma chip.

Not an easy thing to do, but absolutely necessary.

And sometimes, **when the storm clouds clear and the sun shines brightly once again, and that positive momentum puts the wind at your back, you just might be taken on a journey to the edge of paradise with a soul mate who the Universe knew you deserved,** and wanted you to live happily ever after with all along.

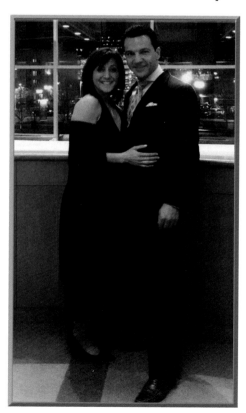

You might already have your soul mate. If so, **good for you my friend.**

If you don't, **you're still on that journey** whether you know it or not. **Enjoy the ride!**

In my case, her name might be **"Dr. Jill" Garripoli.** I'd affectionately refer to her as **"Dr. Feelgood"** because of all the positive mojo she radiates.

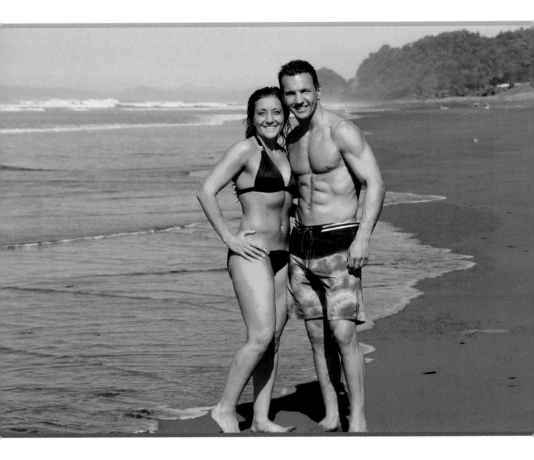

She just might be an award-winning pediatrician **from a big, loud, and loving Italian family whose fairytale dream fits seamlessly into my idea of happily ever after.**

She might actually **enjoy celebrating life** as much as I do and might already have her own admirable version of **the "all in" lifestyle.**

Together, as **a team**, the **vibrant-synergy** we produce might be enough to get me to paradise faster than I ever thought possible.

And maybe, ***just maybe*** … she'll come into my life **without any drama** or baggage, because **that's how "she rolls."**

Nahh … that stuff only happens in the movies. Right?

A Note of Gratitude

Dad and Lynn

Mom and Al

Mike Walter

Randy Bartlett

Neen James

Matt Radicelli

Jim Cerone

Dave Kotinski

Greg Lassik

Wendy Robinson

Richard Bélair

Norma Kahn

Rich Janniello

Brian Snyder

Jeffrey Gitomer

Dr. Jill Garripoli

Your insightful feedback, editing assistance,
and helpful contributions were greatly appreciated.

Thank you for sharing your precious time and talent with me.

Additional Resources

A good book is like a VIP. Your life becomes better after you meet one. The list below features a few of my favorite books that span the genres of wellness, productivity, business management, financial guidance, hospitality, and social media.

Aspire by Kevin Hall
www.powerofwords.com

Book Yourself Solid by Michael Port
www.michaelport.com

Delivering Happiness by Tony Hsieh
www.twitter.com/tonyhsieh

*Doctor's Orders – A Short Guide To A Long Life
by David Agus, MD*
www.davidagus.com

Financial Peace by Dave Ramsey
www.daveramsey.com

Folding Time by Neen James
www.neenjames.com

From Good To Great by Jim Collins
www.jimcollins.com

Little Platinum Book of Cha-Ching by Jeffrey Gitomer
www.gitomer.com

The Gifts of Imperfection by Brene Brown
www.brenebrown.com

The Good Life Rules by Bryan Dodge
www.bryandodge.com

The Purple Cow by Seth Godin
www.sethgodin.com

The Richest Man In Babylon by George S. Clayson
http://tinyurl.com/Inno8ay

The Thank You Economy by Gary Vaynerchuk
www.garyvaynerchuk.com

The World Is Flat – Thomas L. Friedman
www.thomaslfriedman.com

Setting The Table by Danny Meyer
www.twitter.com/dhmeyer

10 Things You Can Do To Have A Better Day by Mike Walter
www.djmikewalter.com

"A book is a device to ignite the imagination."

—ALAN BENNETT

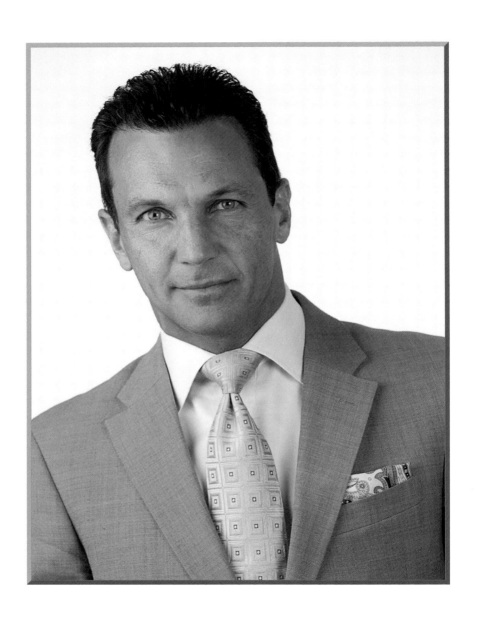

Most people don't spend enough time celebrating their life.

I'd like to help you celebrate yours.

As a lifestyle consultant, I advise individuals, groups, and organizations who are looking to enhance their current fitness, style, and over-all wellness status.

If you or your company would like to schedule a private workshop or speaking engagement on how to live it up, discover fulfillment, and experience the joy you deserve, call (732) 547-1677 or e-mail Mmp@MmpEntertainment.com for pricing, availability, and bookings.

Cheers,

Marcello